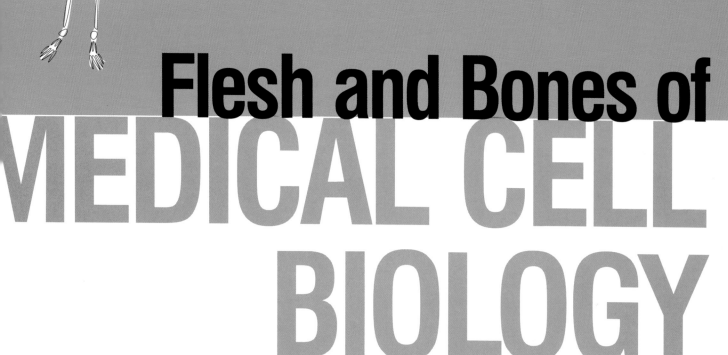

Flesh and Bones of
MEDICAL CELL BIOLOGY

Robert I. Norman BSc PhD
Senior Lecturer in Medical Biochemistry,
Department of Cardiovascular Sciences,
University of Leicester, UK

David Lodwick BSc PhD
Lecturer in Molecular Biology,
Department of Cardiovascular Sciences,
University of Leicester, UK

Illustrations by Robin Dean

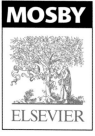

MOSBY

ELSEVIER

Edinburgh   London   New York   Oxford   Philadelphia   St Louis   Sydney   Toronto   2007

First published 2007

ISBN-13: 978-0-7234-3367-5
ISBN-10: 0-7234-3367-4

British Library Cataloguing in Publication Data
A catalogue record for this book is available from the British Library

Library of Congress Cataloging in Publication Data
A catalog record for this book is available from the Library of Congress

Notice
Neither the Publisher nor the Authors assume any responsibility for
any loss or injury and/or damage to persons or property arising out of
or related to any use of the material contained in this book. It is the
responsibility of the treating practitioner, relying on independent
expertise and knowledge of the patient, to determine the best
treatment and method of application for the patient.
The Publisher

Printed in China

The
publisher's
policy is to use
**paper manufactured
from sustainable forests**

Working together to grow
libraries in developing countries

www.elsevier.com | www.bookaid.org | www.sabre.org

ELSEVIER   BOOK AID
            International   Sabre Foundation

your source for books,
journals and multimedia
in the health sciences
www.elsevierhealth.com

Flesh and Bones of
MEDICAL CELL BIOLOGY

Commissioning Editor: **Timothy Horne**
Development Editor: **Barbara Simmons**
Copy Editor: **Jane Ward**
Project Manager: **Frances Affleck**
Designer: **Jayne Jones**

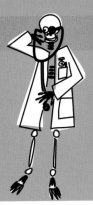

Contents

Cell damage and death

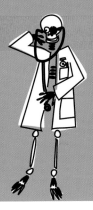

Acknowledgements

We gratefully acknowledge permission for the use of the following artwork:

Electron micrographs in Figs 3.1.1, 3.1.2, 3.1.3, 3.2.2, 3.3.2, 3.31.1, 3.36.2, 3.39.1 and 3.39.3 courtesy of Mrs Evaline Roberts and Dr Arthur J. Rowe.
Electron micrograph in Fig. 3.34.1 courtesy of Dr Jim Norman.

Fig. 3.19.2 from Rettig J, Heinemann SH, Wunder F, Lorra C, Parcej DN, Dolly JO, Pongs O 1994 Nature 369: 289–294, MacMillan Magazines Ltd, Fig. 2.
Fig. 3.40.3 from Harris AK 1994 International Review of Cytology 80: 35–68, Academic Press Ltd, Fig. 4.
Fig. 3.42.3 from Professor A. Kornberg.

The big picture

The key to understanding cell biology is to consider the cell as a large collection of integrated structures and functions, and tissues as a collection of different cell types with different specializations. The biology of all cells is based upon a common set of underlying principles regardless of specialization. It is essential for activities within the cell to be integrated to produce a concerted response to its environment, which will include being responsive to the demands and stimuli of the surrounding tissue.

The occurrence of a common set of underlying principles upon which the biology of all cells is based allows a general picture to be drawn that pertains to any cell of interest. To understand cell biology is to grasp the individual principles and to see them in the context of the integration of structure and function in a whole cell. It is important to remember that cells do not exist in isolation in the human body; rather they are organized into tissues, which often contain a range of different cell types with different specializations. In this context, it is important for a cell not only to integrate its activities within itself to produce a concerted response to its environment but also to be responsive to the demands and stimuli of the tissue in which it is located.

■ THE CELL

The cell is the fundamental unit of life. Any cell is a discrete collection of chemical entities that has the ability to self-replicate.

To be able to reproduce itself, a cell must be able to convert chemicals and energy from its environment into new constituents to permit growth and cell division. This requires the cell to isolate its chemical environment from that of its surroundings so that it can have independent control, **homeostasis** (Fig. 1.1). To achieve such control, cellular contents are enclosed by a cell membrane that is highly impermeable to water-soluble chemicals, thereby preventing ready exchange of chemicals with the environment. Exceptions to this general rule are nutrients and waste materials. Import and export of these chemicals is facilitated by the insertion of specific transporter proteins, which confer selective permeability to the cell membrane. It is also important for viability that a cell can make appropriate responses and adaptations to changes in the external environment. To this end, cell membranes also contain receptor molecules that can recognize external stimuli and the transducing and effector proteins

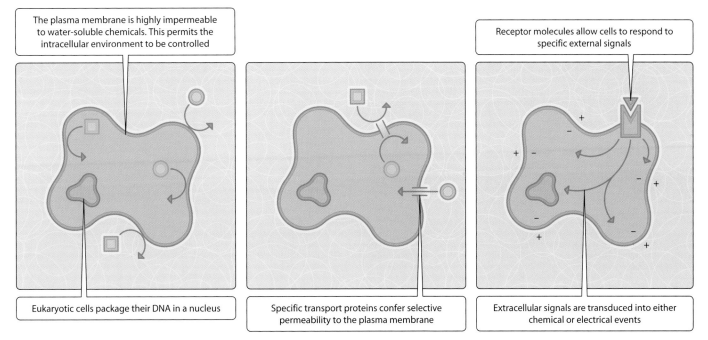

The plasma membrane is highly impermeable to water-soluble chemicals. This permits the intracellular environment to be controlled

Receptor molecules allow cells to respond to specific external signals

Eukaryotic cells package their DNA in a nucleus

Specific transport proteins confer selective permeability to the plasma membrane

Extracellular signals are transduced into either chemical or electrical events

Fig. 1.1 The cell achieves internal homeostasis by controlling passage of molecules through the plasma membrane and by responding to stimuli.

necessary to convert these signals into intracellular events that can modulate the intracellular chemical environment. Responses may be either chemical or electrical.

Genetic information

Although there is an incredible diversity of cell types, the basis of cell structure and function in all cells is surprisingly similar. The information specifying the genetic blueprint for a cell or organism is contained in coded form within the sequence of four different nucleotides within genomic deoxyribonucleic acid (DNA) molecules. The information is divided into units, called genes, each of which encodes a defined protein component (Fig. 1.2). To allow the cell to use the information, single genes are copied or transcribed into smaller related molecules of ribonucleic acid (RNA). The genetic information is then decoded, or translated, from RNA molecules to direct the synthesis of protein molecules. Groups of three nucleotides (triplets) each specify one of 20 different amino acids, such that the nucleotide sequence in the RNA specifies exactly the sequence of amino acids in the translated protein. The amino acid sequences of translated proteins fold into distinct structures prescribed by the amino acids they contain, such that the two-dimensional code of a gene is translated faithfully into a three-dimensional protein structure. The distinct structures adopted by protein molecules define their function. Some proteins are structural components upon which other cellular functions are built. Most often, protein structures define catalytic sites in enzymes that permit cellular biochemical reactions to proceed at appropriate rates under physiological conditions. Yet others form specialized functional molecules, such as ion channels or molecular motors. In this way, the genetic code is translated to provide the full range of specific functionality necessary to define the cell.

Cell types

In the simplest of cells, all constituents, including the DNA, are contained within a single cytoplasmic compartment bounded by the cell membrane. Cells that do not contain a nucleus are termed **prokaryotes** and are generally single-celled organisms. Cells that package their DNA into an organelle enveloped by a double membrane, the nucleus, are termed **eukaryotes**. Some eukaryotic organisms exist as a single-celled organism (e.g. yeast) but most are multicellular assemblies. Once present in an assembly, eukaryotic cells may take on specialized functions to contribute to the benefit of the whole colony. In higher organisms, only the germline cells retain the function of reproduction of the species and the majority of cell types play more specialized supportive roles.

Compartmentalization

In addition to a nucleus, eukaryotic cells also contain a range of other membrane-enclosed structures, or organelles (Fig. 1.3). The subcompartmentalization of eukaryotic cells is the key to the complexity of function that can be achieved by a single cell. By packaging specific activities into discrete membrane-enclosed organelles, cellular processes can be kept separated from each other and can be regulated independently, if necess-

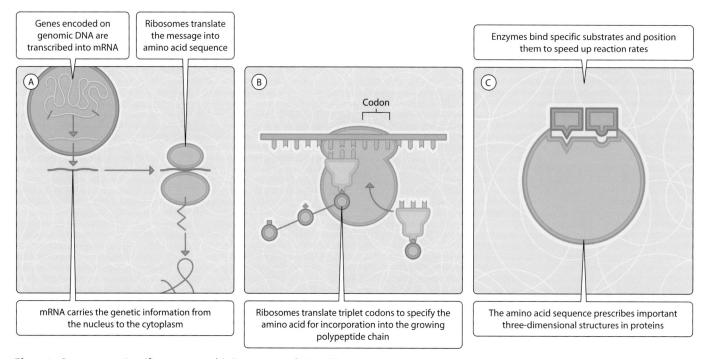

Genes encoded on genomic DNA are transcribed into mRNA

Ribosomes translate the message into amino acid sequence

Enzymes bind specific substrates and position them to speed up reaction rates

Codon

mRNA carries the genetic information from the nucleus to the cytoplasm

Ribosomes translate triplet codons to specify the amino acid for incorporation into the growing polypeptide chain

The amino acid sequence prescribes important three-dimensional structures in proteins

Fig. 1.2 Gene expression (first two panels). Enzyme regulation (C).

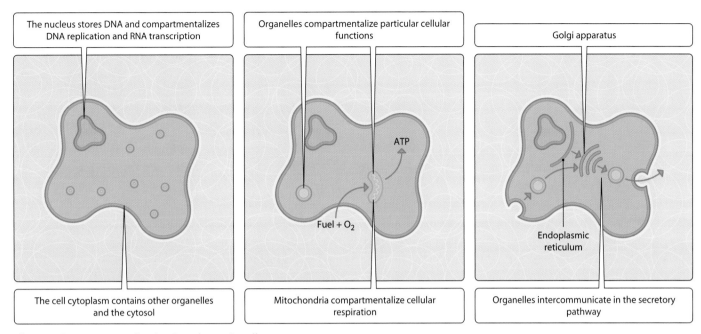

Fig. 1.3 Compartmentalization in eukaryotic cells.

ary. Paradoxically, if the cell is to function as a unit of biology, there must also be extensive communication between different compartments and processes to ensure that a unified and appropriate cellular response is made to the external environment and changing conditions. For this reason, when considering the activity of different components in cell biology, it is always important to remember that they form part of an integrated whole.

Organelles

In somatic cells, in addition to storing two highly condensed copies of the genomic DNA, the nucleus compartmentalizes the reactions of DNA replication and RNA transcription. Ribosome assembly is further compartmentalized to a suborganelle of the nucleus, the **nucleolus**. The nucleus is by far the largest organelle in eukaryotic cells but a range of other organelles also occur within the cell cytoplasm. A second organelle with a double membrane is the **mitochondrion**. This organelle contains its own short DNA molecule encoding 13 proteins and reproduces by division into two. Mitochondria are thought to derive from a symbiotic relationship between a prokaryote and an ancestor eukaryote. The function of mitochondria is to compartmentalize oxidative metabolism and to transfer energy from cell fuels to the production of adenosine 5′-triphosphate (ATP), the energy currency of the cell. Electrons and hydrogen ions removed from fuel molecules are oxidized by molecular oxygen via the electron transport chain in the inner mitochondrial membrane. The energy released is used to drive oxidative phosphorylation of adenosine 5′-diphosphate (ADP) to ATP.

Contiguous with the outer nuclear membrane is the **endoplasmic reticulum** (ER), which forms a series of irregular and interconnected flattened sacs. The ER is a major site of synthesis of cellular components and also those destined for export. It also acts as a centre for detoxification and as an important sink for Ca^{2+}, which when released is important in cellular signalling processes. The **Golgi apparatus** is an organelle consisting of a series of more regularly stacked flattened membrane sacs. This compartment further processes newly synthesized molecules received from the ER. When modifications are complete, the Golgi packages molecules for delivery to other targeted destinations in the cell. One such destination is the **lysosomes**. Lysosomes compartmentalize hydrolytic enzymes, thereby protecting other cellular constituents from inappropriate damage. They are responsible for the digestion of cellular components and those entering the cell by phagocytosis or endocytosis. Other reactions involving molecular oxygen and the production of damaging hydrogen peroxide (H_2O_2) are compartmentalized within **peroxisomes**. Although different organelles carry out different functions, there is considerable transport between organelles, particularly between the ER, Golgi, lysosomes and cell membrane. This is achieved by the budding off of targeted membrane vesicles, which fuse with their targeted organelle and discharge their contents on arrival.

The largest compartment in the cell is the gel-like aqueous environment that remains when all of the organelles are removed, known as the **cytosol**. The cytosol is the site of a large number of cellular chemical reactions. For example, early steps in catabolic (breakdown) pathways are contained in the cytosol (e.g. the breakdown of glucose to pyruvate by the glycolytic pathway). The cytosol also contains ribosomes, the structures on which protein synthesis against the RNA template strand is accomplished.

CELLULAR SIGNALLING

In a multicellular organism, it is important that individual cells act in a concerted fashion to the benefit of the whole. Communication between adjacent cells may be mediated by direct communication of cell cytoplasm through gap junctions, which permit diffusion of small solutes, or by the release of short-lived, local (**paracrine**) signalling molecules to elicit a concerted response from cells in the same tissue (Fig. 1.4). In the nervous system, specialized junctions between neurons, called **synapses**, localize the release of signalling transmitter and the recognition of the signal in the postsynaptic cell. Signalling between cells that are more disparately distributed in the organism may be achieved using hormones. In this case, specialized cells in endocrine glands release hormone into the circulation, where it is transported to the target tissue to bring about a response. Responses to activating and inhibitory stimuli are integrated by the cell so that an appropriate overall response is made.

For a cell to be able to respond to a chemical signal it must display receptor proteins that specifically recognize the signalling molecule and are activated to bring about a change within the cell. A range of strategies is employed to transduce extra-cellular signals into intracellular events. Most often, receptor stimulation at the cell membrane results in the activation of a transducing protein, which, in turn, stimulates an effector enzyme or ion channel within the cell. Effector enzyme activation results in conversion of an inert substrate into an active second messenger, which diffuses through the cytoplasm to activate downstream enzymes or intracellular receptors to bring about a cellular response. In some cases, receptors may be linked directly to ion channels, allowing the external signal to be transduced into an electrical event on the cell membrane. Where signalling is mediated by hydrophobic hormones, such as thyroid hormone, the hormone can enter the cell directly and activate receptors located in the cytoplasm or nucleus; these go on to bind nuclear DNA and regulate gene expression.

In electrically excitable cells, such as nerve fibres and muscle cells, extracellular stimulation can result in a change in potential across the plasma membrane. The membrane potential of resting cells is maintained in a polarized state, negative inside relative to outside, by the equilibration of ions across the plasma membrane. A change in permeability for an ion through channels in the plasma membrane can disturb the resting membrane potential. For example, opening of Na^+ channels results in the influx of Na^+ down the electrochemical gradient. This has the effect of depolarizing the membrane potential and is the basis of the action potential of nerve cells. Propagation of action potentials along a nerve fibre membrane allows nerve impulses to be carried along a nerve axon.

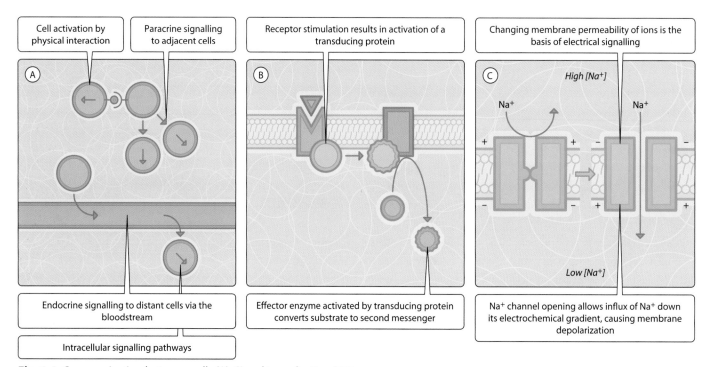

Fig. 1.4 Communication between cells (A). Signal transduction (B,C).

SPATIAL ORGANIZATION WITHIN CELLS

Rather than existing simply as a membrane-enclosed bag of organelles and cytosol, the cell has a much more defined structure. This is determined by a series of protein filaments that combine to form a three-dimensional mesh-like structure, known as the **cytoskeleton** (Fig. 1.5). Cytoskeletal proteins may form attachments with the cell membrane at specific attachment sites or may radiate from near the nucleus. Three main types of filament are employed: thin, intermediate or large diameter. Thin filaments comprise largely the protein actin and are involved in structures in which the generation of contractile forces is involved. Although present in all eukaryotic cells, actin filaments are particularly abundant in muscle cells, where they are further organized into bundles with other contractile proteins. The large-diameter filaments form tube-like structures and so are known as **microtubules**. These structures are particularly important in forming tracks within cells along which membrane vesicles can be directionally targeted to cellular destinations. They are also important in dividing cells as they form the mitotic spindle along which the separation of chromosomes is driven. Microtubules are also found in the specialized structures in cilia and flagella. Here, the relative movement of adjacent microtubules forms the basis of the stroke of cilia or flagella. The intermediate filaments, with diameters between those of the actin microfilaments and microtubules, are a family of proteins that form coiled coils. This group of proteins forms the basis of the tensile strength of the cytoskeleton and provides mechanical stability to the cell overall.

CELL ADHESION AND THE FORMATION OF TISSUES

In higher organisms, the aggregation of cells into tissues allows them to specialize in support of the whole individual. To maintain structural integrity in tissues and to allow a tissue to respond in a concerted manner, the interactions between cells become important. A number of specialized junctional structures form between cells themselves and between cells and the extracellular matrix to anchor them in position within the tissue. Many of these connections also permit communication, for example solute exchange between cells through gap junctions, and the intracellular signal pathway activation by interaction of adhesion proteins. The binding of adhesion proteins within cell–cell and cell–matrix interactions is not static. The strength of adhesion in many interactions may be modulated by the activation of intracellular signalling pathways. These may be activated by chemoattractants or cytokines or may equally be activated by the interaction of adhesion proteins themselves. Thus, cell contacts may make and break in a coordinated fashion, allowing individual cells to migrate within tissues. This is important, for example, in the infiltration of leukocytes and macrophages during inflammatory responses in tissues.

CELL REPLICATION

For a cell to self-replicate it must duplicate its cellular contents, in particular its genetic complement, and must divide into two identical daughter (diploid) cells in a coordinated manner. The process of cell division is cyclical and passes unidirectionally through a series of phases (Fig. 1.6).

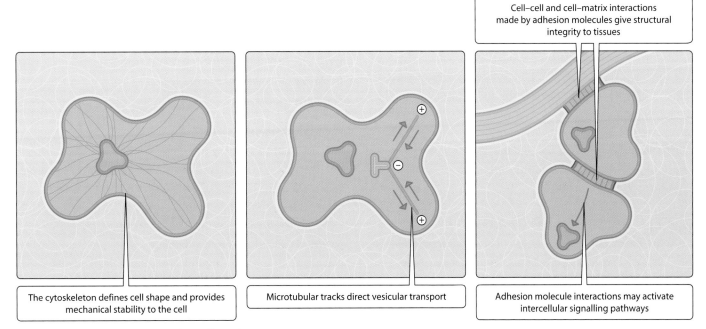

Cell–cell and cell–matrix interactions made by adhesion molecules give structural integrity to tissues

The cytoskeleton defines cell shape and provides mechanical stability to the cell

Microtubular tracks direct vesicular transport

Adhesion molecule interactions may activate intercellular signalling pathways

Fig. 1.5 Spatial organization within cells and tissues.

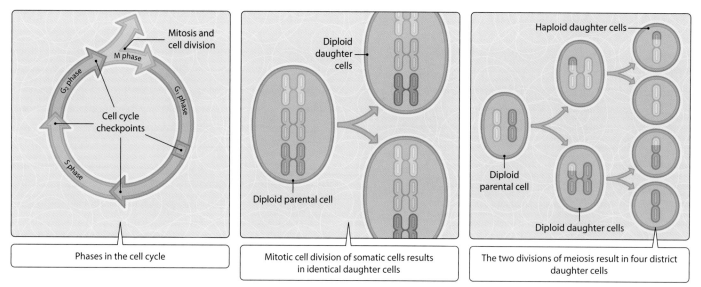

Fig. 1.6 Cell cycle and cell division.

After a period of rapid biosynthesis and growth, the genomic DNA is duplicated and condensed, ready for the separation of paired chromosomes. In **mitosis**, the paired chromosomes are separated to opposite ends of the cell on a mitotic spindle before the cell divides to form two new daughter cells. The cell cycle is controlled at several checkpoints. This allows the cycle of cell division to be arrested if, for example, the nutritional status of the cell is low or if the cell has suffered DNA damage, to prevent replication of damaged DNA.

Gametogenesis and reproduction

In the production of oocytes and spermatozoa, the resulting haploid cells contain only half of the normal chromosome complement of diploid progenitor cells. This is achieved by two cycles of reductive cell division: **meiosis**. In the first cycle, crossing over occurs between paired chromosomes to increase the genetic diversity of the daughter cells. In the second cycle, there is no DNA replication and so sister chromatids separate, resulting in a single copy of each chromosome in each daughter cell. On fertilization of an oocyte, a copy of each chromosome is provided by both gametes and the normal diploid complement is restored.

■ CELL DAMAGE AND DEATH

Cells are always at risk of damage. This may occur following production of damaging chemicals during chemical reactions. In particular, the production of reactive oxygen species during normal metabolism or in response to extracellular challenges can damage cellular constituents, leading to loss of function and necrotic cell death. In order to afford some protection, cells express chemicals and enzymes to inactivate these reactive species. Inevitably some damage occurs, and where this is to DNA there are particular risks for the cell. If a mutation results in altered control of the cell cycle, the cell may become transformed or cancerous and begin to divide in an uncontrolled fashion. Similarly, errors in DNA replication during cell division can have the same result. Cells continually screen for damaged DNA and possess mechanisms to arrest the cell cycle to prevent the replication of damaged DNA and to permit time for DNA repair; however, there is always a danger that cells will escape this check. In some instances, apoptotic cell death is required to allow a tissue to remove cells predestined to become cancerous or to remodel in response to physiological challenge. This occurs via a series of programmed intracellular responses such as the activation of proteolytic caspase enzymes. Inappropriate initiation of apoptosis may contribute to degenerative diseases.

■ SUMMARY

This section has outlined the principles of cell biology. Section two identifies 50 high return facts that form its core concepts and underlying principles. They are the bare bones that will focus your learning and provide an overview on which to build an understanding of cell biology. In Section three, each high return fact is fleshed out in a double-page spread to add further detail and clinical context to the core principle. Students able to learn the 50 facts with some of the fleshed out detail should have no significant gaps in their understanding of the principal workings of a cell and should have a good foundation for more detailed studies in this area.

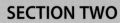

High return facts

The cell

1 Eukaryotic cells range between 10 and 100 μm in length. The genetic material is packaged in the membrane-bounded nucleus. Other membrane-bounded structures, termed organelles, compartmentalize cellular functions and permit greater cellular specialization and diversity.

Organelles

2 Nuclei and mitochondria are both organelles with double membranes. The nucleus is involved in the storage and expression of genetic material; it contains two complete copies of the genomic DNA packaged as chromosomes. Mitochondria are involved in the release of energy from catabolism of fuel molecules as cellular energy currency; consequently, there are more in active tissues. The components of the electron transport chain and oxidative phosphorylation are located on the inner mitochondrial membrane. Mitochondria also contain DNA coding for 13 proteins. This DNA has a maternal pattern of inheritance as the sperm only contributes its nuclear material at fertilization.

3 Single membrane organelles have important roles in secretory and membrane protein biosynthesis, lipid biosynthesis and Ca^{2+} storage (endoplasmic/sarcoplasmic reticulum), protein modification (Golgi apparatus) and cellular digestion (lysosomes).

Genetic information

4 The genetic blueprint for the cell is carried by deoxyribonucleic acid (DNA) a polymer of four repeating chemicals called nucleotides. Chromosomes are made from two strands of DNA, intertwined to produce a double helix. DNA is organized into functional units, called genes. Within each gene are sequences that direct its expression, as well as sequences that describe the structure of the protein product itself. The bases that code for protein are read in threes, each triplet (codon) specifying the incorporation of a different amino acid. Before the information contained within the sequence of DNA can be turned into protein, it must be copied into messenger ribonucleic acid (mRNA), a process called transcription.

5 The coding information in many eukaryotic genes is organized into cassettes (exons) interrupted by regions of junk sequence called introns. Introns are removed from mRNA by splicing. Splicing provides an opportunity to increase the diversity of protein products by controlling whether or not individual exons are retained in the mature message. Amino acids attach to transfer RNAs, which carry a triplet sequence (anticodon) that is complementary to the codon specified by the mRNA. The binding of codon and anticodon brings amino acids in the correct order for assembly into a new polypeptide chain on the ribosome.

Proteins

6 Proteins are composed of a linear sequence of amino acids linked by peptide bonds, with each protein type encoded by a specific gene. Protein structure can be described as primary (linear sequence of amino acids in the polypeptide chain and the position of covalent links between chains), secondary (folding and stabilization into regular structural elements, e.g. α-helix and β-sheet), tertiary (folding and stabilization of segments of secondary structure into a three-dimensional shape and any chemical prosthetic groups) and quaternary (interaction of distinct polypeptide chains into oligomeric complexes). Protein molecules define the specific structural and functional characteristics of cells, functioning as structural proteins, receptors and enzymes.

7 Misfolded or damaged proteins are potentially harmful to the cell. Degradation signals tell the cell which proteins to remove. These proteins are modified by covalent addition of ubiquitin, which targets them for degradation by proteasomes.

Biological membranes

8 Biological membranes comprise a phospholipid bilayer with associated proteins; the proteins may penetrate the bilayer or be associated with one side. Membranes permit enclosed environments to be formed (compartmentalization) and mediate information flow between these compartments (communication).

9 Biosynthesis of secretory and membrane proteins begins on ribosomes in the cytoplasm. Recognition of a newly synthesized N-terminal signal sequence by a signal recognition particle arrests synthesis. Interaction of the signal recognition particle with its receptor on the endoplasmic reticulum allows protein synthesis to recommence; nascent protein is directed into the lumen of the endoplasmic reticulum through a protein translocator complex.

10 Non-polar molecules, such as O_2, CO_2, N_2, urea and, importantly, water, are able to dissolve in and diffuse across the hydrophobic domain of lipid bilayers, whereas the diffusion of ions and small hydrophilic molecules is not favoured. Movement of ions and hydrophilic molecules across biological membranes is mediated by specific membrane transport systems or channels. Transport processes may occur spontaneously (passive transport) or may be driven by the input of energy (active transport).

11 ATP-dependent ion pumps and ion exchangers play important roles in maintaining cellular ion concentrations and, thereby, provide the basis for the regulation of many cellular processes. Ion pumps derive the energy to transport ions across membranes against their electrochemical gradient by using the energy of ATP hydrolysis directly. Exchangers use energy from the movement of one ion down its electrochemical gradient to move another ion or molecule up its gradient.

12 Transmembrane ion transport contributes to the regulation of intracellular pH, volume and nutrient uptake. In the plasma membrane, the energy for these processes is often derived from the inward electrochemical gradient for Na^+. Anion exchange in red blood cells is responsible for their buffering capacity and contributes to their ability to transport O_2 and CO_2 in the circulation. Transport mechanisms for Na^+ in the kidney play an important role in the regulation of circulating Na^+ concentrations.

13 Proteins are targeted either to specific cellular destinations by structural signals within the protein or to a default destination in the absence of a specific signal. Secretory proteins enter either a constitutive (e.g. extracellular matrix proteins) or a regulated (e.g. insulin) secretory pathway.

14 Mature proteins are transported into mitochondria and nuclei via complex ATP-driven mechanisms. Proteins must be unfolded before translocation into mitochondria can commence and cytosolic chaperone proteins help to stabilize the unfolded protein during transfer. Transfer to the nucleoplasm from the cytoplasm occurs through selective nuclear pore structures in the nuclear envelope.

15 Internalization of particulate matter (phagocytosis) and solutes (pinocytosis) occurs by invagination of the plasma membrane to form transport vesicles. Transport between organellar compartments is achieved by the budding off of transport vesicles and movement of these to their destination. Transport vesicle formation is driven by the association of coat proteins, and correct targeting of a transport vesicle is achieved by 'targeting molecules' (SNAREs) in both the transport vesicles (vSNAREs) themselves and the cognate target organelle (tSNAREs). Both vesicle budding and vesicle fusion are governed by small GTP-binding regulatory proteins.

16 Substances too large to enter cells via carrier transport proteins may enter, bound to specific receptors, via receptor-mediated endocytosis. Functions of receptor-mediated endocytosis include metabolite uptake, protein turnover, receptor desensitization and transcellular transport.

Electrical signalling

17 All cells have an electrical potential difference across their plasma membrane (membrane potential); this is expressed as the voltage inside relative to that on the outside of the membrane. The resting membrane potential is established predominantly by the selective permeability of the plasma membrane to K^+, which exits cells through voltage-insensitive K^+ channels until electrochemical equilibrium is reached.

18 Changes in the permeability of a membrane to particular ions (Na^+, K^+, Ca^{2+}, Cl^-) results in a change in the membrane potential and is the basis of electrical signalling. In electrically excitable cells, electrical signals are encoded and propagated in action potentials. In the initial depolarizing phase of the action potential, Na^+ enters the cell through the opening of voltage-gated Na^+ channels. During the repolarization phase, Na^+ channels inactivate and slowly activating K^+ channels open, resulting in the efflux of K^+ and repolarization of the membrane.

19 Ion channels permit the gated movement of ions across membranes in the direction of the electrochemical gradient. Channels may be open constitutively or may be gated by the binding of a ligand or by a voltage change across the membrane. Accessory subunits can alter the kinetic properties of the channel and help to target and anchor it. Mutations affecting channel or accessory proteins are involved in a number of disorders (e.g. cystic fibrosis).

20 Conduction of a nerve impulse is achieved by local currents induced by an action potential in an active region of membrane, which raise adjacent resting regions of the nerve membrane to threshold for firing of an action potential. Myelination of nerves, by decreasing the electrical capacitance of the membrane, speeds up nerve impulse conduction by permitting salutatory conduction where action potentials fire only at nodes of Ranvier. Retrograde conduction of a nerve impulse is prevented by inactivation of ion channels, which makes the nerve refractory to further action potentials until the membrane is reprimed by repolarization.

Chemical signalling

21 For a cell to respond to any chemical messenger, it must produce specific receptor proteins that recognize and produce a response to the signalling molecule. Interaction of the signalling molecule with its specific receptor must then result in the activation of a cellular process; this often involves an amplification cascade. Intercellular chemical signals can be hormones, local mediators or neurotransmitters. A receptor protein is functionally silent unless activated by interaction with an agonist. Binding of an antagonist prevents the action of agonist molecules.

22 Receptors are classified according to the specific physiological signalling molecule (agonist) that they recognize (e.g. acetylcholine receptors). Further subclassification is made on the basis of their ability to be selectively activated by agonist molecules (e.g. nicotinic and muscarinic types). Subclassification is also often made on the basis of the affinity (a measure of tightness of binding) of a series of antagonists. Receptor families

employ a variety of mechanisms to transduce agonist binding into a cellular event, (e.g. integral ion channel, integral enzyme activity, coupling to effectors through transducing proteins, regulation of gene expression).

23 Many membrane-bound receptors employ intermediary proteins to transduce the events of receptor activation to effector molecules in the cell. Agonist-induced conformational changes in the receptor are transmitted to transducing proteins on the cytoplasmic face of the plasma membrane, which then activate the first effector(s) of intracellular signalling pathway cascades. Examples of transducing proteins include insulin receptor substrates (IRS-1) and GTP-binding regulatory proteins (G-proteins).

24 In many instances, the response to receptor activation is the activation of an enzyme effector, which produces a small intracellular messenger molecule or 'second messenger'. Second messengers are normally maintained at low concentration, are produced only in response to specific receptor activation in proportion to the size of the signal and are degraded rapidly to ensure transiency in signalling pathways.

25 Many cellular responses are controlled by changes in the concentration of cytosolic Ca^{2+} ($[Ca^{2+}]_i$). Cells expend a great deal of energy to maintain extremely low resting $[Ca^{2+}]_i$ by extruding it out of the cell or sequestering it into intracellular vesicular stores. On appropriate stimulation, $[Ca^{2+}]_i$ may be raised by re-entry through plasma membrane channels or by release from intracellular stores.

26 Regulation of enzyme and protein activity is often achieved by phosphorylation or dephosphorylation: the directed covalent modification of the protein by the transfer onto or removal of a phosphate moiety, respectively. Protein phosphorylation is catalysed by a family of protein kinases that transfer the terminal phosphate from ATP onto the target residue. Dephosphorylation is catalysed by a family of protein phosphatases that facilitate the hydrolysis of the phosphate bond. There is considerable cross-talk between signalling pathways, which allows pathways to modulate each other and enables an integrated response to extracellular signals.

27 When cells are exposed continuously to an extracellular messenger or drug, they can often become increasingly resistant to stimulation. This loss of sensitivity is known as desensitization or tachyphylaxis when it occurs acutely over a few minutes and tolerance or resistance when occurring over a period of days or weeks.

Integration of signalling mechanisms

28 Transmission of information between excitable cells commonly occurs at specialized junctions called synapses. In response to depolarization and the resulting influx of Ca^{2+}, a chemical neurotransmitter is released from the presynaptic structure of the signalling cell. The neurotransmitter molecule diffuses across the synaptic cleft, binds to a specific receptor molecule on the postsynaptic cell and elicits a response in the postsynaptic cell.

29 Stimulus–secretion coupling in beta-cells of the islets of Langerhans is mediated by ATP-sensitive K^+ (K_{ATP}) channels, which close in response to ATP generated during glucose metabolism; a specialized glucose transporter ensures that the glucose concentration in the cell, and hence the ATP generated, reflects the plasma glucose levels. The resulting membrane depolarization results in Ca^{2+} influx through voltage-sensitive Ca^{2+} channels and stimulation of the insulin secretory machinery.

Cell adhesion

30 The development and function of tissues is dependent on the physical interaction of one cell with another. These physical interactions are mediated by members of several families of membrane-spanning proteins, called adhesion molecules. Adhesion molecules also play important roles in more transient interactions between cells, including those involved in cellular migration and the interactions between cells of the immune system.

31 Many of the cells of the body are grouped together to form tissues, structures or organs, where they function collectively. In order to maintain the structural integrity of tissues and to help individual cells to function in an organized and concerted manner, adhesion molecules on one cell link to similar molecules on adjacent cells, or to the extracellular matrix, forming cellular junctions of differing properties.

32 Much of the human body is made up of connective tissue, which contains few cells and is chiefly made from extracellular matrix; this is a mass of specialized proteins and polysaccharides mainly secreted by fibroblasts. It is the extracellular matrix that gives connective tissue the ability to resist shear, tensile and pressure forces.

33 The extracellular matrix does not simply provide a protective framework; it also has a profound influence on the behaviour of individual cells. The extracellular matrix imparts spatial information that is crucial for development, differentiation, normal cellular function and resistance to apoptosis.

The cytoskeleton

34 The cytoskeleton is a complex dynamic framework of structural protein filaments that defines the shape of a cell and contributes to changes in cell shape and organelle and cell movement. Microfilaments and microtubules are formed from globular actin and tubulin subunits, respectively. They can be rapidly assembled and disassembled as required by the cell.

35 Filamentous protein strands form the structural basis of cell cytoskeletons and contribute to the mechanical stability of cells. Although a heterogeneous group of proteins is involved, each type of filament is composed of a defined protein or combination of proteins.

36 In contractile muscle cells, the cytoskeleton is modified to provide the contractile machinery. Shortening in muscle cells is mediated by the progressive overlap of interdigitated thick and thin filaments composed predominantly of myosin and actin, respectively.

37 Stimulating action potentials are transmitted rapidly deep into skeletal muscle fibres by transverse tubules formed from specialized regions of the sarcolemma. The t-tubular L-type Ca^{2+} channels act as voltage sensors and transmit information physically to ryanodine-sensitive Ca^{2+} channels in the sarcoplasmic reticulum. These channels open to release Ca^{2+} over the sarcomere structures that will initiate contraction. Different muscles types have modifications of this basic method.

38 Transport of organelles and membrane-bound vesicles in eukaryotic cells is directed along 'tracks' of single microtubules by a 'walking' mechanism. The molecular motors for this movement are myosin-like ATPases. Kinesin drives movement from the (−)-end (centrosome end) of the microtubule to the (+)-end, while cytoplasmic dynein drives movement in the opposite direction.

39 Microfilamentous actomyosin structures also occur in non-muscle cells where contractile properties are required (e.g. in cellular locomotion and in the cell cycle to form the contractile ring). Microvilli increase the surface area of epithelial tissues by folding the apical membrane into numerous finger-like projections. Cilia and flagella are specialized surface appendages of cells that have a beating function.

Cell locomotion

40 Cell locomotion is important for a range of processes including infiltration of tissues by specialized cells in inflammation and immunity, fertilization, embryological development and tissue repair and turnover. The forward movement of cells is driven by the 'treadmilling' of actin microfilaments.

Cell division

41 The process of cell division is cyclical and unidirectional. The period between successive divisions is termed interphase; this begins with a period of rapid biosynthesis and cell growth (gap, G_1 phase). Cells can enter a resting phase (G_0) before moving into G_1. After G_1, there is a period when the complete genomic DNA is duplicated (S phase), a second gap phase (G_2 phase), then the division of nuclear material (mitosis) and cytoplasmic division (cytokinesis; M phase with mitosis). Progression through the cell cycle is controlled at 'checkpoints' between stages.

42 DNA replication occurs in the 5' to 3' direction against a 3' to 5' template strand and is initiated by synthesis of a short strand of RNA, which acts as a primer for DNA polymerase. To ensure that the whole genome is replicated within a short time period, DNA is divided into replicons, each with a replication fork; these are activated in clusters.

43 The cell cycle may be arrested at two points (G_1–S and G_2–M) if DNA is damaged. Unrepaired damage can lead to mutation and loss of information so cells express several enzymes that can repair damaged DNA before it is replicated.

44 Mitosis is cell division that produces two diploid cells (containing two copies of each chromosome) from a diploid progenitor cell and occurs in dividing somatic cells. This form of cell division is employed to permit normal growth and repair of all tissues apart from cells involved in the production of gametes.

45 Meiosis is a specialized form of cell division that produces four genetically distinct haploid cells (containing only a single copy of each chromosome) from a diploid progenitor cell (containing two copies of each chromosome). This reductive form of cell division is found only in gamete production: oogenesis and spermatogenesis.

46 The fusion of egg and sperm at fertilization, and the mixing of their haploid genomes, restores the diploid genotype in the resulting zygote. Interaction of sperm with the zona pellucida of the oocyte causes a massive influx of Ca^{2+} and activation of hydrolytic enzymes, which facilitate fusion of the gametes. On fusion, enzymes released from cortical granules modify the zona pellucida to prevent the penetration of further sperm.

47 A cancer is the uncontrolled growth and division of cells that have escaped the normal regulatory mechanisms of the cell cycle. Cancers arise because of mutations in the genome of somatic cells as a result of inaccuracies in gene replication or chromosomal rearrangement at mitosis. Oncogenes are modified genes that result in the loss of host cell growth control. Proto-oncogenes are local host cell genes that normally do not have oncogenic or transforming properties but are involved in the regulation or differentiation of cell growth. If they are disrupted, they can alter control of key regulatory genes leading to unregulated cell division.

Cell damage and death

48 Free radicals are highly reactive species that produce a range of damaging modifications to cellular molecules and thereby contribute to a wide range of disease processes. Normally, cells are protected from excessive free radical damage by the presence of dietary free radical scavengers or antioxidants (e.g. vitamins C and E), the expression of a variety of enzymes (e.g. catalase, superoxide dismutase) and the production of redox active chemicals (e.g. glutathione).

49 Two types of cell death can be distinguished. 'Accidental' cell death or necrosis occurs after severe and sudden injury. It is characterized by the swelling of organelles, loss of the integrity of the plasma membrane and leakage of cellular contents. This leads to an inflammatory response. Programmed cell death or apoptosis occurs in response to physiological triggers in development (tissue remodelling), defence, homeostasis and ageing. It is a controlled dismantling of the cell leading to small apoptotic vesicles, which are then engulfed and digested by macrophages.

50 Most cells in an adult are terminally differentiated. However, we develop from a single cell, so early embryonic cells must have the potential to become any adult cell type. Undifferentiated cells like these are called stem cells. Many adult tissues may also contain cells with the potential to differentiate into one of a limited range of cell types (oligopotent stem cells). The ability to use stem cells to replace or repair damaged or diseased tissues would offer hope for the treatment of many disorders.

Fleshed out

It is very important to have a good understanding of the key cellular structures, their functions and their contributions to the normal internal workings of a cell. Disturbance or dysfunction of cellular mechanisms, such as the homeostasis of metabolite levels, growth, adhesion, chemical and electrical responses to stimuli, movement, adaptation, division and cell death, contribute to many disease processes.

The chapters that follow are presented as double-page spreads, each covering a single high return fact from Section two in more detail. Each chapter is designed to provide an accessible starting point from which the key principles of cellular mechanisms may be understood and learned. These chapters also form succinct revision aids. The questions at the start of each chapter in Section three emphasize the important features of each topic. Cartoon-strip illustrations are used in every chapter to illustrate the more difficult concepts and the medical relevance of topics is highlighted by discussion of related clinical conditions in boxed text. It is important to note that emphasis in this section is on human and animal cell biology, although molecular principles are often similar in prokaryotic cells. As you build up your knowledge from these chapters, you should find it easier to obtain more detailed information from more complex texts and information sources.

1. Cellular organization

Questions
- Why are cells necessary to biology?
- What is the main difference between prokaryotic and eukaryotic cells?
- Why are organelles necessary in eukaryotic cells?

The cell: the unit of biology

The cell is the smallest functional unit of living organisms and tissues. Cellular contents are delineated by a selectively permeable plasma membrane, which permits control over the internal environment. Cells are classified as prokaryotic or eukaryotic on the basis of the absence or presence of a nucleus, respectively.

Prokaryotic cells

Prokaryotic cells, represented by bacteria, are relatively small (1–5 μm in length) simple cells that contain some subcellular structures but are essentially devoid of discrete intracellular membrane-bounded organellar structures (Fig. 3.1.1). All of the cellular contents, including the single circular genomic deoxyribonucleic acid (DNA) molecule, are contained within the cytoplasm. Often, prokaryotic cells are surrounded by a protective cross-linked lattice that forms a cell wall.

Eukaryotic cells

Eukaryotic cells of higher organisms, including humans, are larger than prokaryotic cells, ranging between 10 and 100 μm in

length. In addition to the packaging of multiple linear strands of DNA in the membrane-bounded nucleus, eukaryotic cells contain other membrane-bounded structures, termed **organelles**, which compartmentalize cellular functions and permit greater cellular specialization and diversity (Fig. 3.1.2). Even in the cytoplasm, there is a degree of molecular compartmentalization. A complex cross-linked network of structural proteins extends from specialized contacts in the plasma membrane, involved in cell-cell and cell-substratum interactions, to dense structures surrounding the cell nucleus, this is known as the intracellular **cytoskeleton**. It acts to maintain the basic cell shape and also has important dynamic functions, contributing to cellular processes such as the movement of organelles, endocytosis, secretion and cell division. The cytoskeleton also allows the cytoplasm to be subdivided into microcompartments, by restricting free Brownian diffusion; this may help to localize individual enzymes catalysing sequential reactions into the same cell regions such that metabolites may be channelled from one enzyme to the next, increasing the efficiency of catalysis.

The cytosol is the largest compartment in eukaryotic cells and constitutes about half the cell volume. It contains water and dissolved ions, metabolites, building blocks, proteins and ribonucleic acids (RNAs) and is the location of many metabolic pathways.

Viruses

Viruses are non-cellular, prokaryotic lifeforms that are obligate parasites (i.e. they are incapable of replicating without the assistance of a host cell). Viruses have a simple structure with a

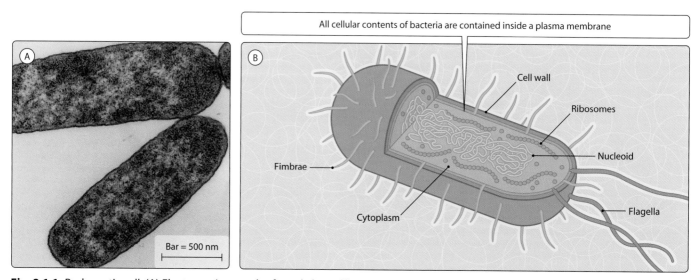

All cellular contents of bacteria are contained inside a plasma membrane

Cell wall

Ribosomes

Nucleoid

Fimbrae

Flagella

Cytoplasm

Bar = 500 nm

Fig. 3.1.1 Prokaryotic cell. (A) Electron micrograph of a rod-shaped bacterium (e.g. *Escherichia coli*); (B) the basic cell structure.

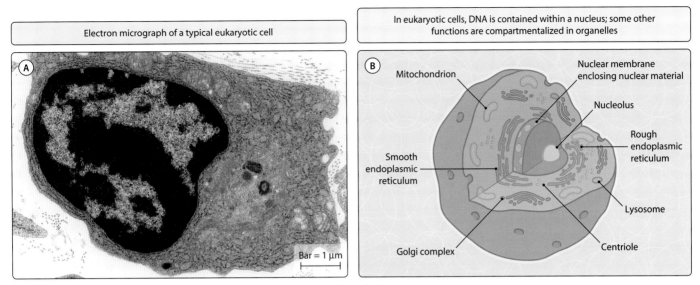

Fig. 3.1.2 Eukaryotic cell. (A) Electron micrograph of a typical cell; (B) the basic cell structure.

DNA or RNA genome enclosed in a protein shell or capsid (made up of self-assembling capsid proteins) (Fig. 3.1.3). Some viruses also have an envelope of lipid bilayer membrane, which they acquire when leaving the host cell by budding. Surface proteins are recognized by receptor proteins on host cells and allow the viral particle to be taken up into the cell by receptor-mediated endocytosis (Ch. 16) for replication.

Prions

Prions are non-cellular, proteinaceous, infectious agents. They are not lifeforms in their own right but have the ability to disrupt normal cell function leading to disease. Prions are misshapen forms of an endogenous protein that can invade cells and interact with normal copies of the protein, converting them into the prion form. A number of neurodegenerative diseases may be caused by prions; the most notable being new variant Creutzfeldt–Jakob disease.

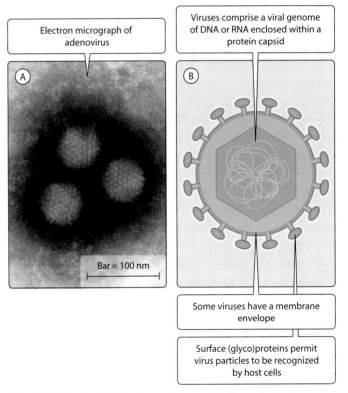

Fig. 3.1.3 A virus. (A) Electron micrograph of an adenovirus; (B) the basic structure.

2. Organelles with double membranes

Questions
- What cellular functions does the nucleus perform?
- How is nuclear DNA packaged in a non-dividing eukaryotic cell?
- Why is it important that the inner mitochondrial membrane is essentially impermeable to protons?

The nucleus

With the exception of mature red blood cells and platelets, every eukaryotic cell contains a nucleus (8 μm diameter) (Fig. 3.2.1). The nuclear matrix or nucleoplasm contains two complete copies of the genomic DNA, which in non-dividing cells (interphase) is packaged into chromosomes. The chromosomal complement or karyotype of normal humans is 22 homologous pairs of chromosomes plus the sex chromosome pair XY in males and XX in females. The nuclear envelope consists of a double-layer membrane separated by the periplasmic space. The outer nuclear membrane forms a continuum with the rough endoplasmic reticulum (ER) and the periplasm forms a continuum with the ER lumen. The structure of the nucleus is determined by the nuclear lamina, a dense network of rod-like lamin neurofilaments that forms associations between DNA molecules and the inner membrane.

The nucleus compartmentalizes reactions involving the synthesis of DNA, RNA and ribonuclear protein complexes. This permits the post-transcriptional processing of mRNA before translation into protein in the cytoplasm. A suborganelle of the nucleus is the **nucleolus**, in which new ribosomes are assembled.

Chromatin

In non-dividing cells, the single molecule of double-stranded DNA that makes up each chromosome is packaged into a dense and highly organized supercoiled structure of DNA, protein and some RNA, called chromatin. In interphase, the highly condensed form, termed heterochromatin, is localized around the periphery of the nucleus. In interphase, approximately 10% of the chromatin is in the unwound form (euchromatin) to permit gene transcription to occur.

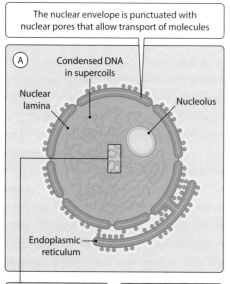

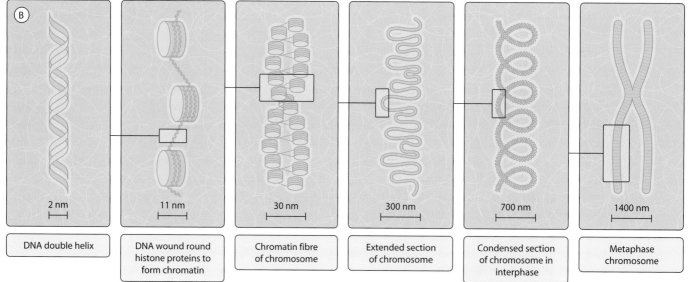

2 nm	11 nm	30 nm	300 nm	700 nm	1400 nm
DNA double helix	DNA wound round histone proteins to form chromatin	Chromatin fibre of chromosome	Extended section of chromosome	Condensed section of chromosome in interphase	Metaphase chromosome

Fig. 3.2.1 The nucleus. (A) Cross-section of a typical nucleus in interphase; (B) DNA in a chromatin supercoil.

Mitochondria

Mitochondria provide the machinery for oxidative phosphorylation, which allows the efficient release of energy from catabolism of fuel molecules and the concomitant production of the cellular energy currency, adenosine 5′-triphosphate (ATP). Enzymes of the major metabolic pathways (citric acid cycle, fatty acid β-oxidation) are located in the matrix, while the components of the electron transport chain and oxidative phosphorylation are all located on the inner mitochondrial membrane. Mitochondria are, therefore, more prevalent in active tissues and are often localized within cells at sites of cellular activity. These ellipsoid organelles (2–3 μm × 0.5–1 μm) are coated by a smooth outer membrane that is punctuated with transmembranous porin pores, which allow the passage of proteins up to ≈ 10 kDa (Fig. 3.2.2). Thus, for small molecules and H⁺ (protons), the intermembrane space is essentially continuous with the cytoplasm. The inner membrane is essentially impermeable to protons and is highly convoluted into cristae, which protrude into the mitochondrial matrix. This permits a gradient of H^+ to be generated across the membrane to drive the synthesis of ATP.

DISEASES MEDIATED BY MITOCHONDRIAL GENES

The mitochondrial genome encodes just two mitochondrial ribosomal RNAs, 22 transfer RNAs (tRNA) and 13 subunit components of the electron transport/oxidative phosphorylation complexes. Mutations here can lead to a number of diseases, but the link between mutation and clinical features is often obscure. Severity of a disease mediated by a mitochondrial gene may be reduced by the presence of non-defective mitochondria, so-called **heteroplasmy**. Mitochondria grow and divide during interphase and are shared between daughter cells on cell division. Because most mitochondrial proteins are encoded in the nucleus, most mitochondrial diseases are inherited in a Mendelian fashion. However, because the sperm only contributes nuclear material to the ovum at fertilization, mutations in mitochondrially encoded proteins have a maternal pattern of inheritance.

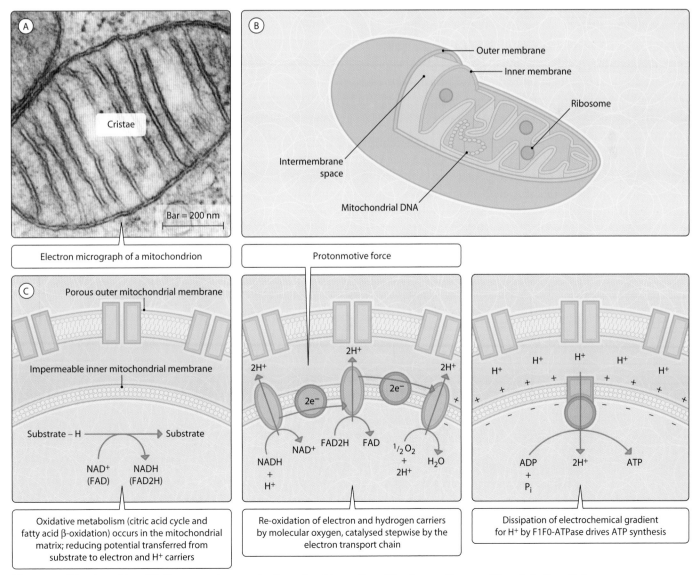

Fig. 3.2.2 Mitochondrion. (A) Electron micrograph of an ultrathin section; (B) cutaway diagram; (C) metabolic activity.

3. Organelles with single membranes

Questions
- What is the difference in function between 'rough' and 'smooth' endoplasmic reticulum?
- What are the functions of the Golgi apparatus?
- Why are lysosomes and peroxisomes important in cellular physiology?

Cells can be disrupted by shear forces in a homogenizer and the components can then be separated by centrifugation.

Endo(sarco)plasmic reticulum

The endoplasmic reticulum (ER), or sarcoplasmic reticulum (SR) in muscle cells, is composed of flattened sacs and tubules (cisternae) of membrane within the cytoplasm and often forms concentric layers around the nucleus. It forms a continuation of the nuclear envelope such that the ER lumen is continuous with the periplasmic space of the nuclear envelope. This membrane structure may represent up to half of the total cell membrane in an actively secreting cell. The association of ribosomes with the ER allows regions of 'rough' ER to be distinguished from areas of smooth ER devoid of ribosomal contacts. Ribosomes associated with rough ER are involved in the synthesis of secretory, lysosomal and membrane proteins. Both rough and smooth ER are involved additionally in: protein glycosylation (Fig. 3.3.1); lipid biosynthesis (membrane lipids, phospholipids, steroids and triglycerides); functions involving electron transport activities, such as the introduction of double bonds into fatty acids by the cytochrome b_5 electron transport chain; detoxification of cellular toxins and drugs by the cytochrome P450 electron transfer system; and the delivery of newly synthesized secretory or membrane proteins to the Golgi apparatus. Regions of the ER take up Ca^{2+} and contribute to the maintenance of low cytoplasmic Ca^{2+} concentration ($[Ca^{2+}]_i$). This store is an important source of Ca^{2+} that can be mobilized for intracellular signalling (Ch. 25).

The Golgi apparatus

The Golgi apparatus (or complex) consists of stacks of flattened smooth membrane sacs and vesicles. A major function of the post-translational modification of secretory and membrane proteins is by sequential glycosylation (Figs 3.3.1 and 3.3.2). The Golgi complex is organized functionally into cis-, median- and trans-Golgi such that distinct modifications are made in each region as a newly synthesized protein moves from the ER through the cis-Golgi (close to the ER) to the trans-Golgi (close to the periphery of the cell). The sorting of newly synthesized membrane proteins to their cellular destination occurs in the trans-Golgi network.

Lysosomes

Lysosomes sequester hydrolytic enzymes in a distinct compartment to protect other cellular components. Primary lysosomes are formed by budding-off from the Golgi complex. Fusion with intracellular vesicles (endosomes) to form secondary lysosomes is important for the breakdown of materials entering the cell by phagocytosis and fluid-phase and receptor-mediated endocytosis.

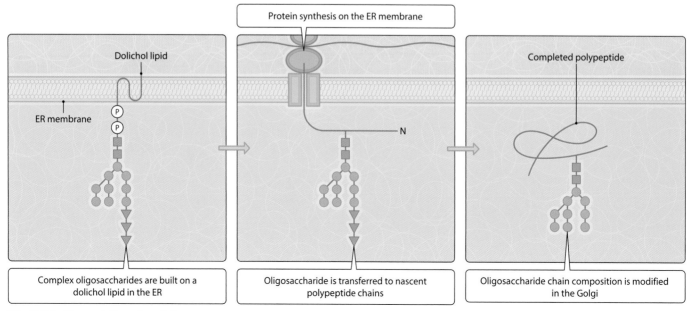

Protein synthesis on the ER membrane

Dolichol lipid

ER membrane

P
P

N

Completed polypeptide

| Complex oligosaccharides are built on a dolichol lipid in the ER | Oligosaccharide is transferred to nascent polypeptide chains | Oligosaccharide chain composition is modified in the Golgi |

Fig. 3.3.1 Glycosylation of proteins.

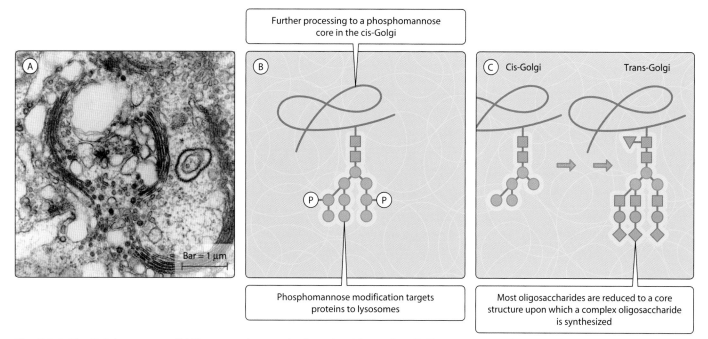

Fig. 3.3.2 The Golgi apparatus. (A) Electron micrograph of an ultrathin section; (B,C) processing in the cis- and trans-Golgi.

Lysosomes also contribute to turnover of cell components (autophagocytosis).

Peroxisomes

Peroxisomes are small organelles that isolate potentially damaging oxidative reactions involving molecular oxygen and resulting in the production of hydrogen peroxide (H_2O_2) and organic peroxides (Ch. 48). They contain abundant catalase (up to 40% of peroxisomal protein), which converts toxic H_2O_2 to oxygen and water. The functions of peroxisomes vary between tissues but include detoxification, the breakdown of long-chain and branched fatty acids, biosynthesis of cholesterol and lipid,

and protection from the accumulation of excess oxalate and purines.

LYSOSOMAL STORAGE DISEASES

Mutations in lysosomal enzymes that result in loss of function or abnormal targeting to the lysosome give rise to the lysosomal storage diseases, with overlapping phenotypes (Fig. 3.3.3). In inclusion cell (I-cell) disease, carbohydrate side-chains lack mannose 6-phosphate, leading to inappropriate sorting of lysosomal enzymes for export. Large undigested inclusion bodies form in the lysosomes and patients develop severe skeletal deformities and psychomotor deficiencies.

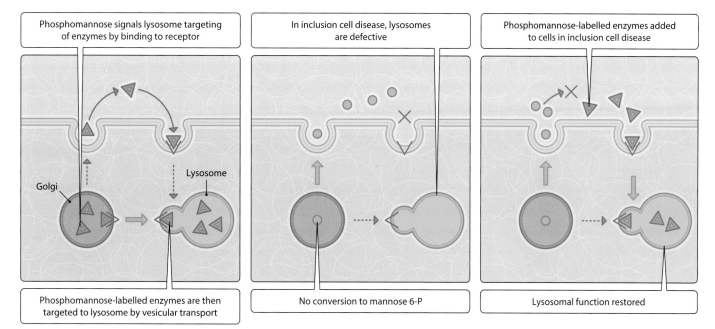

Fig. 3.3.3 Inclusion cell disease.

4. DNA and gene transcription

Questions
- How is genetic information stored in the cell?
- What is the structure of DNA?
- How is gene expression controlled?

DNA and the chromosomes
The genetic blueprint for the cell is carried by DNA, which is a polymer of just four repeating chemicals called nucleotides. The four nucleotides are each composed of unique nitrogen bases (adenine, cytosine, guanine and thymine) and common triphosphate and deoxyribose sugar moieties. The sugar and phosphate groups are linked to one another by phosphodiester bonds to form a DNA molecule. It is the order in which the nucleotides are incorporated into the DNA chain that carries the information. Despite having only four 'letters', this genetic 'alphabet' is sufficient to describe all the 'recipes' necessary to make and maintain a complex organism with thousands of different proteins.

Chromosomes are made from two strands of DNA, intertwined to produce a double helix (Fig. 3.4.1). This structure, in which the two molecules of DNA are arranged head to toe, is stabilized by hydrogen bonding between their respective bases. Adenine (A) pairs specifically with thymine (T) and guanine (G) with cytosine (C) (and vice versa). This specific base pairing means that the two strands of DNA are complementary in base sequence. That is, wherever an A is found in one strand, a T will

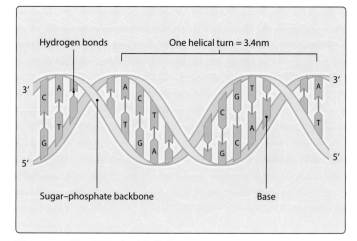

Fig. 3.4.1 The DNA double helix.

be found in the other, and, wherever a G is found, a C will be present in the complementary strand.

The two strands of DNA are described as sense and antisense. The sense strand carries the coding information that describes the final protein, whereas the antisense strand carries the complement of this sequence in the reverse orientation. The information contained in DNA is organized into functional units, called **genes**, each one carrying the instructions for making a single protein. Within each gene are sequences that direct its expression, as well as sequences that describe the structure of the protein product itself (coding sequence). The bases that code for protein are read in threes, each triplet (**codon**) specifying the incorporation of a different amino acid (Fig. 3.4.2).

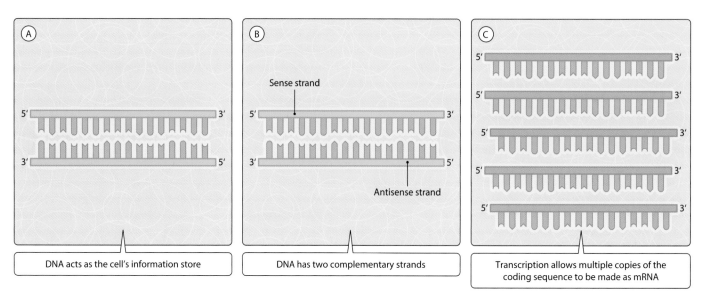

Fig. 3.4.2 Heritable information is stored in DNA.

Before the information contained within the sequence of DNA can be turned into protein, it must be copied into RNA and exported into the cytoplasm. RNA is similar in structure to DNA and binds to it readily, but it contains ribose instead of deoxyribose, does not form a double helix, and uses a fifth base, uracil (U), instead of thymine. This step, which is called **transcription**, allows genes to be read individually (Fig. 3.4.3). The potential to make many RNA copies of a gene also allows the message to be amplified; thus, thousands of copies of a protein can be produced rapidly from a single gene.

Gene expression

Although the genome contains all the information necessary to replicate an organism, proteins are needed in varying amounts, at different times and in different places, each according to its function. Cells must also respond appropriately to external stimuli. Selective expression of genes also explains how a nerve cell and a muscle cell look and act so differently yet share exactly the same set of genes. It appears that this specialization results from differences in expression of relatively few genes. Most genes, such as those required for normal metabolic activities (housekeeping), are expressed at fairly constant rates in all cells.

Transcription

Genes are transcribed by enzymes called **RNA polymerases**, which produce mRNA, an RNA copy of the sense strand of the DNA. Transcription is controlled by the interaction between specific DNA sequence motifs, DNA-binding proteins (**transcription factors**) and RNA polymerase. Genes that need to be regulated together may share binding sites for particular transcription factors, allowing their transcription to be controlled coordinately by the availability of these factors in the cell. Tissue specificity can work in the same way: if a transcription factor is only expressed in a particular cell type then genes that require it will only be expressed in those same cells.

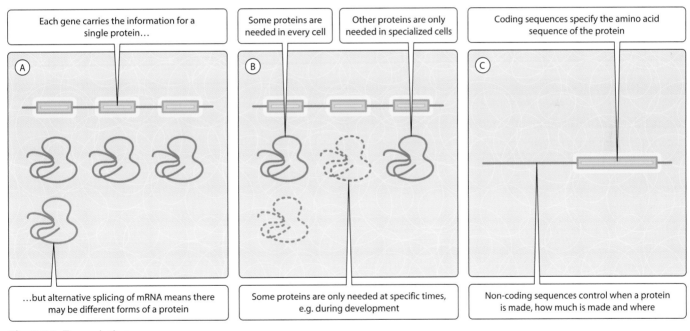

Fig. 3.4.3 Transcription.

5. Messenger RNA and translation

Questions
- How is the information in mRNAs organized?
- How can the cell make more unique proteins than it has genes?
- How do mRNAs direct protein synthesis?

Messenger RNA

The 5′-end of the newly transcribed mRNA molecule is capped with a methylated guanosine residue (Fig. 3.5.1). This cap is added as soon as the RNA polymerase has transcribed the first part of the message and is required both for efficient initiation of translation by the ribosome and for protection of the 5′-end of the growing mRNA from degradation. In eukaryotes, the 3′-end of the message is determined by site-specific cleavage rather than simply by termination of transcription, allowing the mRNA molecule to be varied to produce different protein structures. Once cleavage has occurred, large numbers of adenine residues are added to the end of the transcript to produce a poly-A tail, which protects the mRNA molecule from degradation and acts as a signal for export from the nucleus. Altering the rate at which a gene is transcribed is the most obvious way of controlling the synthesis of its product. However, all the subsequent steps in the path from primary transcript to translated protein (i.e. mRNA processing, export, stability and translation) may also be regulated.

Splicing of mRNA

In prokaryotes, genes are organized as contiguous sequences (i.e. all the code required for making a particular protein is found in an uninterrupted stretch of DNA). In eukaryotes, the coding sequence is often interrupted by 'junk' sequences called **introns**, which are transcribed to RNA along with the coding sequences (**exons**) but then removed from the transcript by a process called splicing; this produces a mature mRNA that can then be translated into protein (Fig. 3.5.2). Splicing can be used to produce different versions of a protein by choosing whether or not to include particular exons in the mature message. Alternative splicing considerably increases the number of different proteins that can be made from a limited set of genes and explains why the human genome contains less genes ($\approx$ 30 000) than was anticipated. The mRNA molecules remain tethered within the nucleus until they are fully matured. Once all these steps have been carried out, the mRNA molecule is ready for export from the nucleus through the nuclear pores into the cytoplasm.

Stability

The rate at which individual mRNA molecules turn over varies between a few minutes and several hours. For genes whose product is required in fairly constant amounts (e.g. housekeeping genes), turnover can be slow, with each mRNA molecule being translated many times over a period of hours. Some renewal of the pool of mRNA molecules is necessary to maintain the integrity of the message. Other genes may need to be induced swiftly in response to an external stimulus but then turned off again rapidly once the need for their product has passed. If these mRNAs persist after the stimulus has been removed then so will the response, which may be detrimental to the cell. One way to avoid this is for these particular mRNA molecules to have a short half-life (i.e. a high rate of turnover).

Translation

The information carried by mRNAs is translated into protein in the cytoplasm by ribosomes, complexes of ribosomal RNA and protein (Fig. 3.5.3). Ribosomes identify the initiation codon

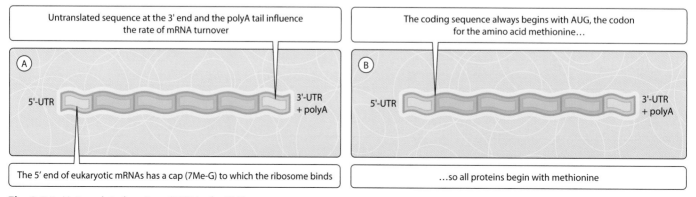

Fig. 3.5.1 Untranslated regions (UTRs) of mRNA.

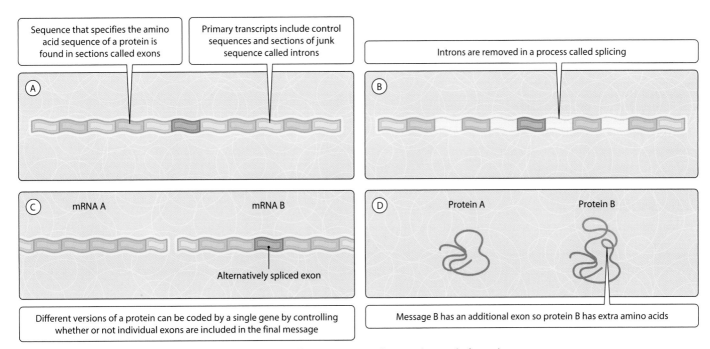

Fig. 3.5.2 Splicing of mRNA increases the number of different proteins that can be made from the genome.

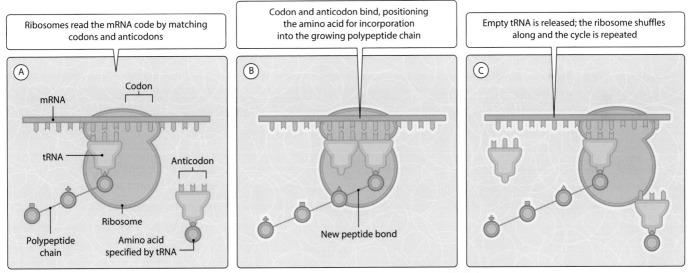

Fig. 3.5.3 Protein synthesis is carried out by complexes of ribosomal RNA and protein called ribosomes.

(AUG) and make a polypeptide chain by linking the amino acids specified by this and the subsequent codons. The amino acids are brought to the ribosome bound to specific RNA molecules called transfer RNAs (tRNAs). These tRNAs carry a triplet sequence (or **anticodon**) that is complementary to the codon specified by the mRNA. By matching codon and anticodon, the ribosome can ensure that it is incorporating the correct amino acid. The codon for the last amino acid of the protein is followed by one of three termination codons, which signal to the ribosome that its job is done.

6. Proteins and protein function

Questions
■ How do proteins confer specificity to cellular functions?
■ What are the levels of protein structure?
■ How can protein activity be regulated?

Protein structure
Protein molecules have defined structures that specify their function and allow them to make highly specific contributions to cellular processes. Proteins are composed of a linear sequence of amino acids (residues) linked by peptide bonds. Each protein is encoded by a specific gene. The genetic code is transferred from the nucleus to the cytoplasm by mRNA, which is translated on ribosomes into protein sequences. Each codon directs the incorporation of one of 20 possible L-amino acids into the growing polypeptide chain (Fig. 3.6.1). Amino acids comprise a central alpha carbon atom linked to an amino group, a carboxyl group, a hydrogen atom and, importantly, a variable R group, which defines the character of the amino acid. A peptide bond (N–C) is formed when an amino and carboxyl group of two amino acids react. The bond is planar owing to its partial double-bond character. This restriction in motion around the axis of the linear sequence of residues, together with steric hindrance between the R groups of adjacent residues, limits the possible structures available to the protein. A specific amino acid sequence, therefore, defines a unique three-dimensional structure and proteins are said to be either **fibrous** (elongated structure, e.g. myosin) or **globular** (highly folded structure, e.g. haemoglobin).

   Protein structure can be described at four levels.

1. *Primary structure*. The linear sequence of amino acids in the polypeptide chain and the position of covalent links between chains (e.g. S–S disulphide bonds).

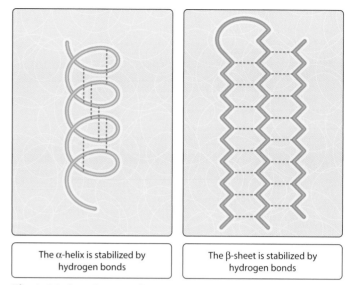

The α-helix is stabilized by hydrogen bonds

The β-sheet is stabilized by hydrogen bonds

Fig. 3.6.2 Protein secondary structure.

2. *Secondary structure*. The folding and stabilization (hydrogen bonds) of the primary structure into regular structural elements (e.g. α-helix and β-sheet) (Fig. 3.6.2).
3. *Tertiary structure*. The folding and stabilization of segments of secondary structure into a three-dimensional shape and the interaction with prosthetic groups (Fig. 3.6.3).
4. *Quaternary structure*. The interaction of distinct polypeptide chains (subunits) to form oligomeric protein complexes.

A genetic mutation resulting in the substitution of one amino acid for another residue may produce significant alterations in the protein's structure and, hence, function.

   Proteins oscillate between different thermodynamically stable structures (conformations). Under extreme conditions (e.g. high temperature, extreme pH and organic solvents), proteins may unfold. Some can refold into their native active structures but often unfolding is irreversible (**denaturation**).

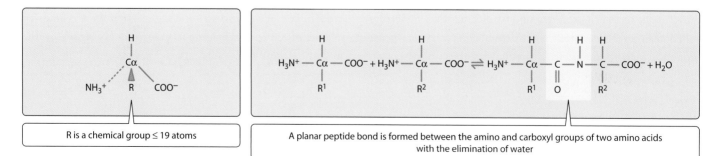

R is a chemical group ≤ 19 atoms

A planar peptide bond is formed between the amino and carboxyl groups of two amino acids with the elimination of water

Fig. 3.6.1 General formula for an L-amino acid at neutral pH and formation of a peptide bond.

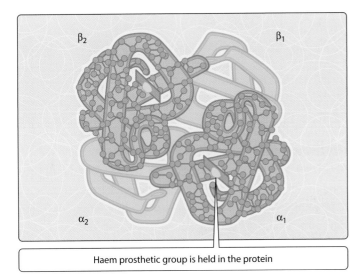

Haem prosthetic group is held in the protein

Fig. 3.6.3 Tertiary and quarternary structure in haemoglobin.

Protein function

The defined spatial positioning of amino acids in protein structures permits the orientation of R groups to form binding sites, or clefts, for chemical groups. The ability to recognize and interact specifically with other chemical entities is fundamental to the function of all proteins. Proteins can be subdivided into three groups:

- structural proteins, which may be either elongated fibrous proteins or globular proteins
- receptor proteins, which transduce the molecular recognition of a chemical moiety into a cellular event (e.g. hormone and neurotransmitter receptors, antibodies in immune recognition)
- globular proteins, which are catalytic (enzymes).

The enzymes are by far the biggest group and provide the microenvironment to accelerate chemical reactions. Enzymes are catalysts; therefore, they are present in the same form at the beginning and end of a reaction. They can catalyse reactions in both the forward and reverse direction depending on the concentration of substrates and products.

Regulation of protein activity

The activity of proteins is often regulated by:

- competitive binding of an inhibitory substance at the active site (competitive inhibition)
- covalent modification of the active site
- activation or inhibition by proteolytic cleavage
- binding of a regulatory (allosteric) molecule at a second site on the protein; this may be inhibitory (non-competitive inhibition) or stimulatory (Fig. 3.6.4)
- covalent modification at an allosteric site independent of the active site; in particular, phosphorylation/dephosphorylation reactions.

The rate of a reaction catalysed by an enzyme will vary with the type of inhibition (Fig. 3.6.5).

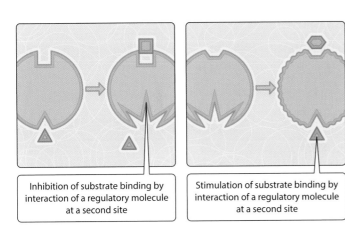

Inhibition of substrate binding by interaction of a regulatory molecule at a second site

Stimulation of substrate binding by interaction of a regulatory molecule at a second site

Fig. 3.6.4 Regulation of protein activity.

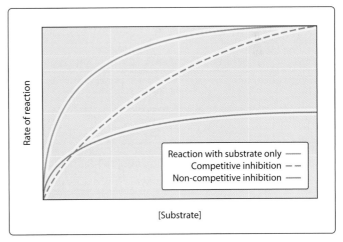

Reaction with substrate only ——
Competitive inhibition – –
Non-competitive inhibition ——

[Substrate]

Fig. 3.6.5 The effect of inhibitors on the rate of an enzyme-catalysed reaction.

7. Proteasomes and protein turnover

Questions
- Why do cells need efficient mechanisms for the disposal of proteins?
- What is the function of proteasomes?
- How do cells prevent all proteins being destroyed by proteasomes?

Damaged proteins

Misfolded or damaged proteins are of no use to a cell and are potentially damaging because they could form inappropriate aggregates with other important macromolecules. Such proteins are quickly destroyed. Proteins generally fold with hydrophilic residues facing the exterior aqueous medium, and hydrophobic residues buried in the core. Misfolding of a protein after synthesis, denaturing damage or an abnormal amino acid side-chain after oxidative damage (Ch. 48) can all reveal inappropriate hydrophobic patches that can address the protein for regulated destruction. Such destruction also allows cells to control the levels of subsets of proteins. Some proteins are degraded rapidly at all times, permitting rapid response to inhibition of gene expression; degradation of others may depend on other conditions in the cell. For example, the cyclins that regulate cell division are generally long lived but are quickly removed when the cell needs to progress to the next stage of the cell cycle (Ch. 41). Degradation signals can be unmasked on regulated proteins by changes in conformation (e.g. subunit dissociation or protein phosphorylation). Turnover rate can also be specified by the nature of the N-terminal residue. Proteolytic removal of the N-terminal residue or a short N-terminal sequence may also accelerate the degradation of an intracellular protein (Fig. 3.7.1).

Proteasomes

Regulated proteolysis is carried out by an abundant, large complex of proteolytic enzymes called the proteasome (Fig. 3.7.1), a large hollow cylinder composed of four rings of seven subunits. A number of these subunits are proteases and their active sites face into the chamber of the cylinder. A large protein cap or gate is associated with each end of the cylinder. The proteasome is responsible for recognition and unfolding of proteins targeted for destruction. Energy for protein unfolding is supplied from ATP hydrolysis by a number of ATPases in the cap complex. Unfolded proteins entering the proteasome are acted upon repetitively until only small peptides and amino acids remain, which are released into the cytosol.

Ubiquitinylation

To avoid all cellular proteins becoming susceptible to proteasomes, proteins for degradation are targeted by modification with multiple copies of a small protein called ubiquitin (Fig. 3.7.2). Ubiquitin is activated by an ubiquitin-activating enzyme (E1) and then transferred to an active site on ubiquitin-conjugating enzyme (E2). Proteins displaying degradation signals are recognized by an accessory protein (E3), which combines with E2 to form ubiquitin ligase. Ubiquitin is then transferred from E2 to a lysine residue on the protein to be degraded.

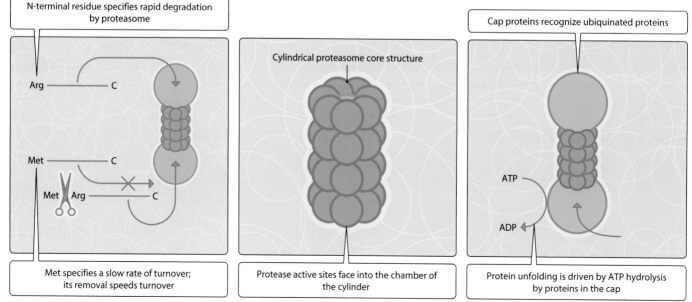

Fig. 3.7.1 Proteasomes.

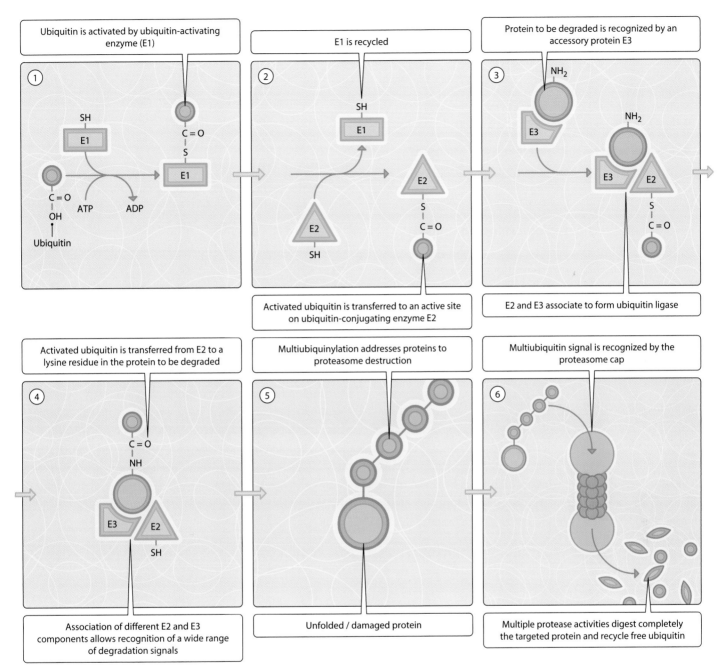

Fig. 3.7.2 Ubiquitinylation.

A multiubiquitin chain is formed by the addition of further ubiquitin molecules, linked through their C-termini to a specific lysine residue within the preceding ubiquitin chain. In humans, multiple forms of E2 and E3 yield a large range of similar but distinct complexes, each recognizing different degradation signals.

ANTIGEN PRESENTATION

Foreign antigens produced on intracellular infection with a pathogen (e.g. virus) are degraded by the ubiquitinylation–proteosome mechanism. Peptides so produced are ultimately presented at the cell surface bound to major histo-compatibility complex class I (MHC I) proteins. Recognition by cytotoxic T cells initiates cell destruction.

NEURODEGENERATIVE DISEASES

When the ubiquitinylation–proteasome mechanism fails, large and damaging protein aggregates form in the affected cell, e.g. neural accumulation of beta-amyloid in Alzheimer's disease, which may contribute to dementia.

8. Membrane structure and dynamics

Questions
- What are the functions of biological membranes?
- How are the lipid components organized in biological membranes?
- How does cholesterol stabilize the plasma membrane?

General functions of biological membranes

Compartmentalization
Biological membranes form a continuous sheet-like barrier around cells or intracellular compartments. By restricting the diffusion of most substances and facilitating the movement of others through a wide variety of protein pores and transport systems, membranes present highly selective permeability barriers that allow the control of the chemical environment in cellular compartments and between the cell and its surroundings.

Communication
Membranes contribute to biological communication by mediating information flow between cellular compartments and between cells and their environment. The presence of specific molecules in membranes allows recognition of stimuli in the form of chemical signals (e.g. hormones, local mediators and neurotransmitters), electrical events (changes in membrane potential) and light (retina) as well as generation of secondary signals, which may be physical, chemical or electrical, in response to recognition of the primary stimulus. Different membranes may have specialized functions.

Membrane structure
The lipid mosaic theory of membrane structure (Singer–Nicholson model) considers biological membranes to be composed of a lipid bilayer with associated membrane proteins, which may be associated with the surface (peripheral proteins) or deeply embedded (integral proteins) in the bilayer (Fig. 3.8.1C). Approximately 40% of the membrane is lipid. These molecules are amphipathic (i.e. they contain both hydrophilic and hydrophobic moieties). Phospholipids are the predominant class of lipids. An enormous variation in phospholipids is possible through the use of a range of polar head groups and fatty acid chains. Other less-abundant amphipathic lipids, such as glycolipids and sphingomyelin, also contribute to the bilayer structure. Membrane proteins, which make up approximately 60% of a biological membrane, carry out the distinctive functions of membranes and include enzymes, transporters, pumps, ion channels, receptors, energy transducers and structural elements. Membrane components often have an asymmetric distribution. Directional orientation of proteins is particularly important for function.

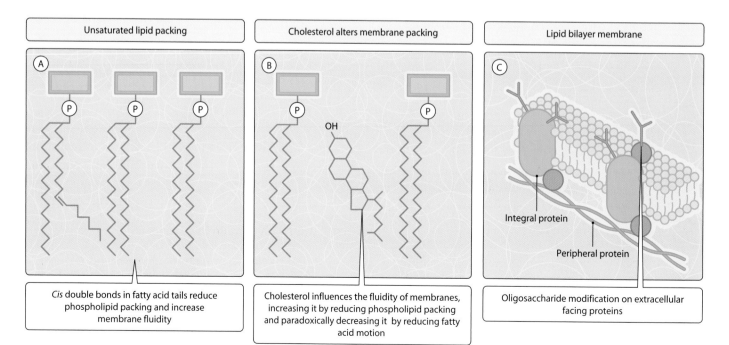

Unsaturated lipid packing	Cholesterol alters membrane packing	Lipid bilayer membrane

Cis double bonds in fatty acid tails reduce phospholipid packing and increase membrane fluidity

Cholesterol influences the fluidity of membranes, increasing it by reducing phospholipid packing and paradoxically decreasing it by reducing fatty acid motion

Oligosaccharide modification on extracellular facing proteins

Fig. 3.8.1 Membrane structure.

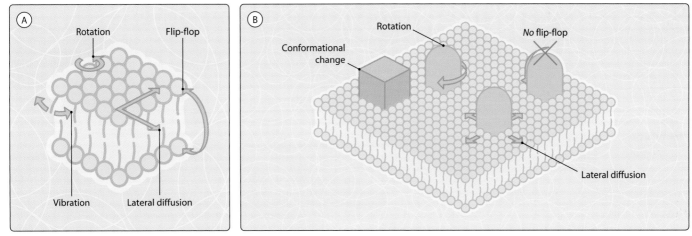

Fig. 3.8.2 Mobility of lipids (A) and proteins (B) in membranes.

Dynamics in lipid bilayers

Membrane bilayers are not fixed structures; rather lipid molecules may vibrate, rotate, move laterally or, occasionally, flip their head group through the hydrophobic domain of the bilayer to the other side (flip-flop) (Fig. 3.8.2). The presence of a double bond in a fatty acid side-chain, which is nearly always in the *cis* conformation in natural lipids, introduces a kink in the aliphatic chain that reduces the ability of the phospholipid to pack in a crystalline array and, therefore, contributes to increased membrane fluidity (Fig. 3.8.1A). These motions result in a fluid, two-dimensional bilayer structure in which considerable movement of constituent molecules can occur. Integral membrane proteins may change conformation, rotate and move laterally, but no flip-flop is permitted because of thermodynamic constraints of moving large hydrophilic groups through the hydrophobic core. Integral membrane proteins tend to separate out into the fluid phase or cholesterol-poor regions, and movement may be further restricted by associations with other membrane proteins and/or extramembranous proteins (peripheral proteins) such as cytoskeletal proteins.

Role of cholesterol in plasma membranes

In plasma membranes, cholesterol is present at almost equimolar concentrations with phospholipids and plays an important role in stabilizing this structure (Fig. 3.8.1B). Molecules of cholesterol are immobilized against adjacent phospholipids through the formation of a hydrogen bond between the hydroxyl group of cholesterol and the carboxyl group of the phospholipid. Paradoxically, the presence of cholesterol reduces phospholipid packing and, hence, maintains the membrane in a fluid phase, while the rigid cholesterol ring structure held close to the fatty acyl chains reduces intrachain vibrational movements, thereby reducing membrane fluidity. Thus, cholesterol contributes to relatively constant dynamic properties of the lipid environment in the plasma membrane.

MEMBRANES IN DISEASE PATHOLOGY

The loss of integrity of normal membrane structure is often associated with disease processes. For example, in diabetes mellitus, insulin receptors and glucose transporters are destroyed in response to inappropriate protein glycosylation caused by hyperglycaemia, thereby contributing to insulin resistance in this condition.

9. Secretory and membrane protein biosynthesis

Questions
- How is biosynthesis of secretory and membrane proteins in the cytoplasm prevented?
- How is membrane protein orientation achieved?
- Where does post-translational modification of secretory and membrane proteins occur?

Biosynthesis

Like cytosolic proteins, membrane proteins and those to be secreted or targeted to lysosomes are synthesized against the mRNA template by ribosomes. However, before synthesis pro-gresses very far, the translation of these proteins is halted until the ribosome has been transferred to the rough endoplasmic reticulum (ER). A characteristic hydrophobic amino acid sequence of 18–30 residues flanked by basic residues at the N-terminus of the nascent polypeptide, termed the signal or leader sequence, is recognized by a large protein–RNA complex called the **signal recognition particle** (SRP) (Fig. 3.9.1). Binding of the SRP to the polypeptide–ribosome complex prevents further protein synthesis while the ribosome is in the cytoplasm.

On the ER, the SRP is recognized by an SRP receptor. This interaction directs the SRP–ribosome complex to interact with a protein translocator complex (Sec61). This releases the SRP

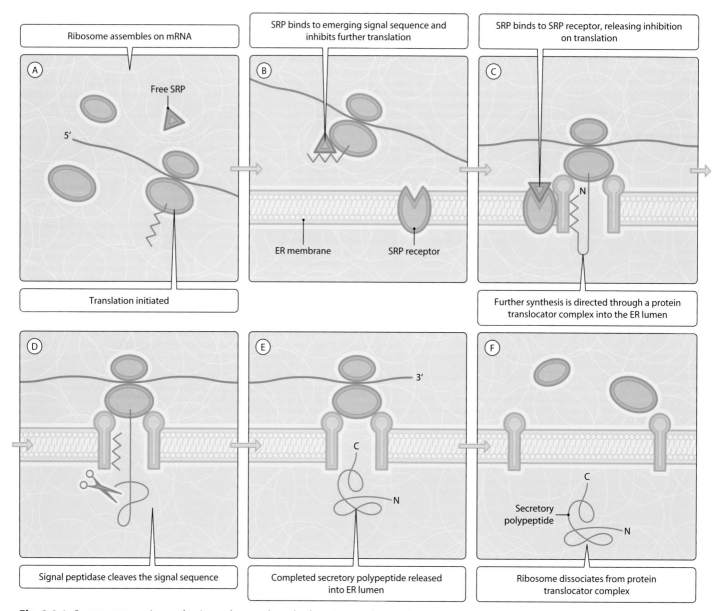

Fig. 3.9.1 Secretory protein synthesis on the rough endoplasmic reticulum (ER).

from the signal sequence of the nascent polypeptide, thereby removing the inhibitory constraint on further translation. Further synthesis is directed through the ER membrane via the pore of the protein translocator. In the case of a secreted or lysosomal protein, the completed protein is extruded into the lumen of the ER. If a segment of hydrophobic sequence occurs in the nascent polypeptide chain, this acts as a stop-transfer signal and arrests the growing polypeptide in the membrane. A lateral gating mechanism releases the membrane protein from the protein translocator. The ribosome then presumably detaches from the ER and protein biosynthesis continues in the cytoplasm. For both secretory proteins and membrane-incorporated proteins, the signal sequence is cleaved from the new protein by signal peptidases even before protein synthesis is completed.

In principle, internal start-transfer sequences may bind to the translocator in either orientation (Fig. 3.9.2). In one orientation with more positive residues at the N-terminus of the start-transfer sequence, the C-terminal section passes into the lumen. Where the more positive residues are at the C-terminal end of the start-transfer sequence, the N-terminus of the nascent protein is translocated. In this case, no signal peptidase cleavage occurs.

Proteins with multiple membrane-spanning domains
Where a protein traverses the membrane repeatedly, the first two transmembrane domains are targeted for insertion via internal start- and stop-transfer sequences, as above. Further start- and stop-transfer sequences reinitiate the translocation of additional hydrophobic domains. Whether all of the trans-membrane domains are aggregated within the protein translocator complex during synthesis and released into the membrane together or inserted into the membrane sequentially during synthesis has not been resolved.

Insertion of membrane proteins synthesized in the cytoplasm
A few membrane proteins that are synthesized totally in the cytoplasm, including all mitochondrial proteins, can be inserted post-translationally into membranes by an ATP-driven process. Stabilizing chaperonin proteins and tunnel-forming proteins in the membrane are probably involved. Some proteins become membrane anchored via a post-translational covalent addition of a fatty acid (palmityolation, mystriolation), which binds the protein to a single leaflet of the membrane bilayer.

Post-translational modification of secretory and membrane proteins

In addition to signal peptide cleavage, post-translational modifications to secretory and membrane proteins, such as disulphide bond formation, N-linked glycosylation and proteolytic modification, are commenced as soon as the amino acid to bear the modification appears in the lumen of the ER (Ch. 3). The nascent chain is further processed as it passes from the ER and through the cis- to the trans-Golgi, providing a mechanism for an ordered series of modifications. The new protein continues along the secretory pathway until the secretory vesicle fuses with the plasma membrane. At this point, secreted proteins are released from the cell and membrane proteins are delivered such that the regions of the protein that were located in the cytoplasm during synthesis remain with this orientation.

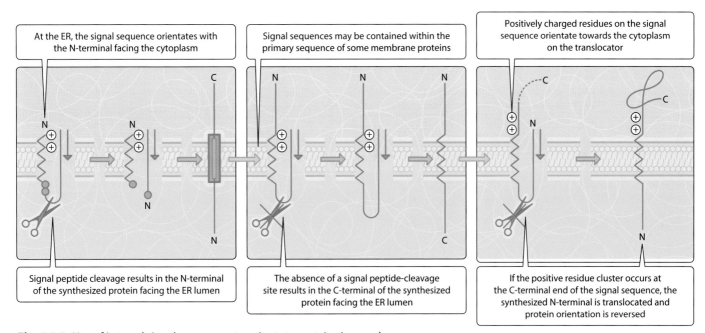

Fig. 3.9.2 Use of internal signal sequences to orientate proteins in membranes.

10. Membrane permeability

Questions
- What molecules are able to diffuse across membrane bilayers freely?
- How do ions and small polar molecules permeate hydrophobic membrane bilayers?
- What is the difference between passive and active transport across membranes?
- What is the difference between primary and secondary active transport?

Diffusion across lipid bilayers
Lipid bilayers are freely permeable to small unchanged molecules (e.g. O_2, CO_2, urea) and hydrophobic molecules (e.g. steroids) but are impermeable to ions and large polar molecules (e.g. glucose, Na^+). Passive transport is linearly related to concentration.

Surprisingly, membranes are relatively permeable to water, which diffuses passively up the concentration gradient of a solute, the osmotic gradient. In some cells (e.g. kidney proximal tubule), the movement of water may be facilitated by specific water channels, called **aquaporins**.

Membranes as permeability barriers
Movement of hydrophilic ions or molecules across the hydrophobic core of an intact biological membrane is a very rare event; hence, membranes act as permeability barriers to all charged and hydrophilic molecules. The movement of molecules and ions across a membrane is mediated, and regulated, by specific membrane transport systems or channels with important roles in many cellular processes (Fig. 3.10.1).

Facilitated diffusion
The presence of specific proteins in a bilayer can substantially increase the permeability of a polar substance (e.g. permeability of Cl^- through a pure phospholipid bilayer is exceedingly low but is ~ 10^7-fold higher through the erythrocyte membrane because an anion transporter (band 3) is present.

Facilitated transport is a saturable process as each carrier can interact with only one or a few ions or molecules at any moment and a finite number of transporters are present in the membrane. Therefore, as the concentration gradient increases, a maximum rate of transport will be reached when all the transporters are 'busy'. As with enzyme catalysis, the maximum rate of transport is greatly enhanced by facilitated transport but the equilibrium point for the transported species is not altered. Some ion-transporting channels may be gated by ligand binding (Chs 22 and 25) or by voltage (Chs 18 and 19).

Active transport
Whether the transport of an ion or molecule can occur spontaneously (passive transport) or requires energy (active transport) is determined by the free energy change of the transported species (Fig. 3.10.2). The free energy change is determined by the concentration gradient for the transported species and by the electrical potential across the membrane bilayer when the transported species is charged. To overcome unfavourable

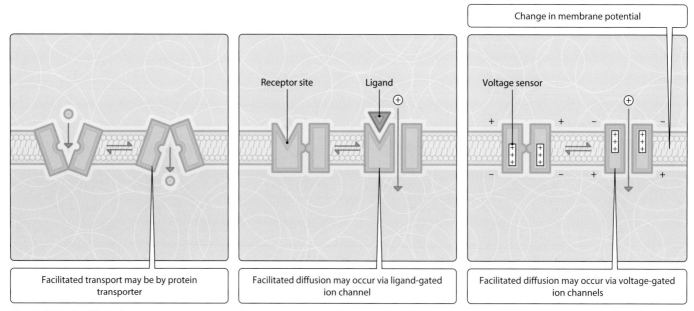

| Facilitated transport may be by protein transporter | Facilitated diffusion may occur via ligand-gated ion channel | Facilitated diffusion may occur via voltage-gated ion channels |

Fig. 3.10.1 Facilitated movement across membranes.

chemical or electrical gradients, movement must be coupled to a thermodynamically favourable reaction (Fig. 3.10.3). The free energy to drive active transport comes from the hydrolysis of ATP, either directly via the activity of ATP-dependent pumps (**ATPases**) in 'primary active transport' or indirectly by 'secondary active transport' processes that use other energy sources. For example, the Na^+–K^+-dependent ATPase (or Na^+ pump) exchanges ions, three Na^+ outwards and two K^+ inwards, against the respective concentration gradients at the expense of one ATP molecule hydrolysed. Running the pump in reverse provides an ATP generator. In mitochondria, dissipation of a gradient of H^+ is used to drive ATP synthesis via an ATP-dependent proton transporter. Secondary active transport may be driven by gradients of substances or ions (often Na^+), light and high-potential electrons, often generated at the expense of ATP hydrolysis.

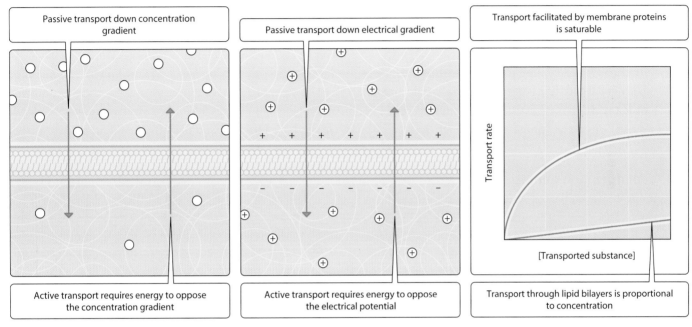

Fig. 3.10.2 Active and passive transport.

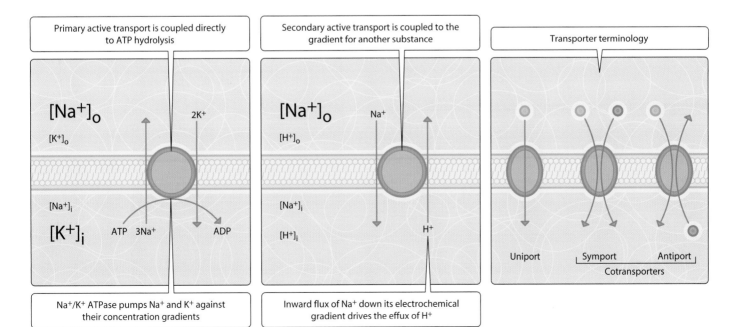

Fig. 3.10.3 Energy for active transport.

11. Ion pumps and ion exchangers

Questions
- What is the normal distribution of ions across the plasma membrane of a resting cell?
- How do the activities of ion pumps and exchangers differ?
- What are the roles of the Na^+/K^+-ATPase in cellular physiology?
- How do transport proteins contribute to the maintenance of a low intracellular Ca^{2+} concentration?

Ion distribution across the plasma membrane
Gradients are maintained (outside/inside) for Na^+ (145/10 mmol/l), K^+ (4.5/160 mmol/l), Ca^{2+} (1.5/< 0.0001 mmol/l) and Cl^- (114/3 mmol/l) across the plasma membrane by the activity of ATP-dependent ion pumps and ion exchangers.

ATP-dependent ion pumps
Ion pumps derive the energy to transport ions across membranes against their electrochemical gradient by using the energy of ATP hydrolysis directly. A number of important ion-transporting ATPases make important contributions to cellular physiology (Fig. 3.11.1 and Ch. 12).

The Na^+/K^+-ATPase or Na^+ pump
The Na^+/K^+-ATPase is found in all cells and is crucial to the maintenance of the gradients for Na^+ and K^+ across the plasma membrane in resting cells. Creation of these gradients is important to provide the driving forces for processes such as the regulation of resting membrane potential (Ch. 17), cell volume, cytoplasmic pH and adsorption through epithelia (Ch. 12). For each ATP hydrolysed, three Na^+ are removed from the cell (efflux) and two K^+ are brought in (influx).

The plasma membrane Ca^{2+}/Mg^{2+}-ATPase
The Ca^{2+}/Mg^{2+}-ATPase in the plasma membrane (Ca^{2+} pump or PMCA) presents a high-affinity mechanism for the active extrusion of Ca^{2+} against the electrochemical gradient, maintaining the low $[Ca^{2+}]_i$ at the expense of ATP hydrolysis. In some cells, such as the erythrocyte and myocardial muscle cells, the binding of Ca^{2+}-calmodulin results in a reduction in the Michaelis constant (K_M) for Ca^{2+} and to an increase in maximum activity of the transporter, allowing cells to react quickly to restore resting $[Ca^{2+}]_i$.

The sarcoplasmic reticulum Ca^{2+}-ATPase
A second Ca^{2+}-ATPase is found in the sarcoplasmic or endoplasmic reticulum (SERCA). This transporter provides for the active transport of Ca^{2+} into vesicular stores in the cell and is an important mechanism in cellular signalling (Ch. 25).

Ion exchangers
Ion exchangers move cations (Fig. 3.11.2) or anions (Fig. 3.11.3). Exchange of anions can be either independent of, or dependent on, the electrochemical gradient for Na^+.

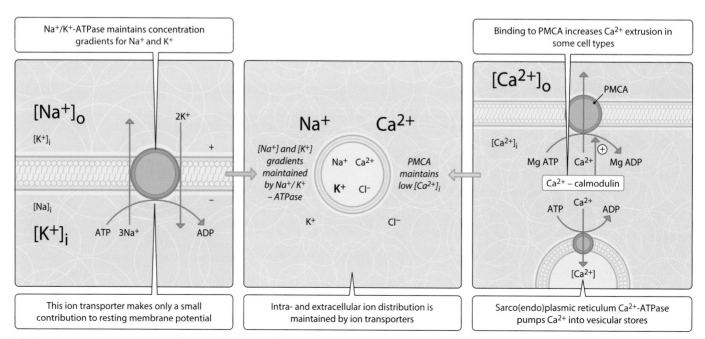

Fig. 3.11.1 Ion-transporting ATPases in ion homeostasis.

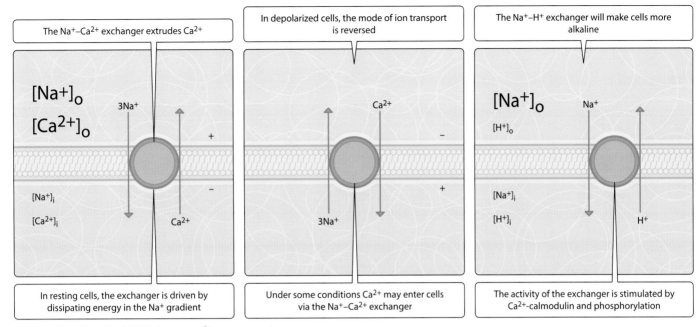

Fig. 3.11.2 Control of cytoplasmic Ca^{2+} concentration.

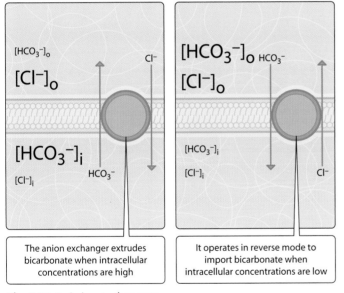

Fig. 3.11.3 Anion exchangers.

The Na⁺–Ca²⁺ exchanger

The Na^+–Ca^{2+} exchanger is a high-capacity, low-affinity secondarily active transport system that extrudes Ca^{2+} from the cell by using energy from the influx of Na^+ down its electrochemical gradient and the membrane potential. This plasma membrane transporter pumps Ca^{2+} out from the cell after cell stimulation when $[Ca^{2+}]_i$ is raised (e.g. in cardiac muscle). One Ca^{2+} is exchanged for the inward movement of three Na^+ and, therefore, the transporter is electrogenic. In depolarized membranes, the Na^+–Ca^{2+} exchanger activity reverses and, thereby, contributes to Ca^{2+} influx (e.g. during the cardiac action potential).

The Na⁺–H⁺ exchanger

The Na^+–H^+ exchanger is a secondarily active exchanger that uses the inward electrochemical gradient for Na^+ to expel H^+ from the cell. It is electroneutral, exchanging one Na^+ for one H^+ across the plasma membrane. This exchanger is present in all cells, can function to regulate cell pH and cell volume and is important in cell growth.

Sodium-independent anion exchanger (Cl⁻–HCO₃⁻ exchanger)

The Na^+-independent Cl^-–HCO_3^- exchanger in the plasma membrane mediates the exchange of one Cl^- for one HCO_3^- and is, therefore, electroneutral. Transport may be in either direction. This transporter can function to load cells with Cl^- against the electrochemical gradient for Cl^- to regulate cell volume and to reduce cell alkalinization by removal of HCO_3^-.

USE OF NA⁺/K⁺-ATPASE INHIBITORS IN THE TREATMENT OF CONGESTIVE HEART FAILURE

Cardiac glycosides (e.g. digoxin, ouabain), which are inhibitors of the Na^+/K^+-ATPase, are used in the treatment of congestive heart failure to reduce Na^+ gradients and, thereby, increase membrane potential, action potential firing and, ultimately, the force of contraction (positive inotropy; Ch.18). Increased cellular Na^+ content also reduces the Ca^{2+} extrusion activity of the Na^+–Ca^{2+} exchanger (see above), resulting in cellular retention of Ca^{2+}, which is sequestered into intracellular stores. Release of this additional stored Ca^{2+} on cardiac excitation (Ch. 37) contributes to the positive inotropism of these agents.

12. Ion transporters in cellular physiology

Questions

- In what ways do membrane transporters contribute to the regulation of pH, cell volume and nutrient uptake?
- How does the action of diuretic drugs in kidney tubules modify urine output ?
- How does anion exchange activity contribute to O_2 loading and delivery by erythrocytes?

Ion transporters maintain ionic concentration gradients and regulate cell pH (Fig. 3.12.1) and volume (Fig. 3.12.2).

Regulation of pH

When the short-term buffering capacity (PO_4^{3-}, HCO_3^- and protein) of a cell is exceeded, pH is controlled by the transport of H^+ and HCO_3^- across the plasma membrane. Most cells possess both Na^+–H^+ exchangers (NHE) and anion exchangers, which extrude H^+ and HCO_3^- from the cell, respectively. Cell acidification activates NHE in most cells and Na^+–Cl^-–HCO_3^-–H^+ counter-transporters and Na^+–HCO_3^- cotransporters, where present. All are driven by inward movement of Na^+, hence Na^+/K^+-ATPase activity is crucial. Cell alkalinization is normally

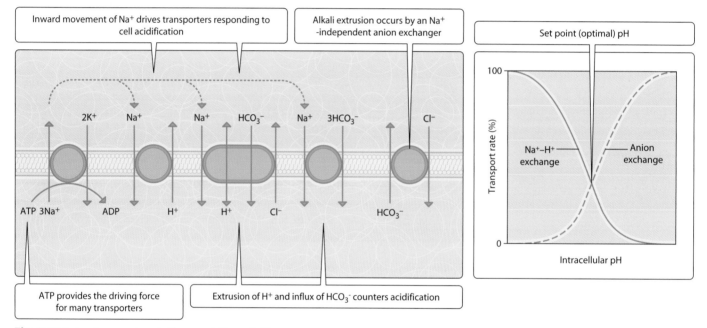

Fig. 3.12.1 Ion transporters in the regulation of pH.

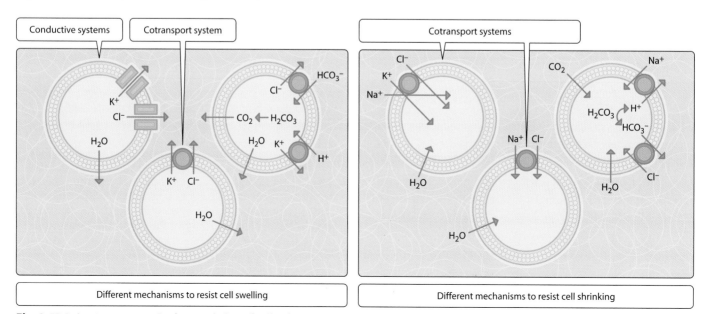

Fig. 3.12.2 Ion transporters in the regulation of cell volume.

controlled by the extrusion of HCO_3^- by Na^+-independent anion exchangers.

Volume regulation

Cell volume changes are mediated by the movement of water across membranes in response to modifications in osmotic strength. Osmotic gradients are altered by the movement of ions (Na^+, K^+ and/or Cl^-) or osmotically active compounds, such as sugars. Na^+/K^+-ATPase maintains a low intracellular Na^+ and provides the driving force for the passive diffusion of K^+ or Cl^- in response to cell swelling and the Na^+–K^+–$2Cl^-$ cotransport system in response to cell shrinking, and/or the concerted action of proton and anion exchangers. In some cells, it appears that swelling-operated channels for efflux of organic solutes may exist (e.g. myoinositol, in the brain, or amino acids).

Transport of small molecules

Transporters that mediate facilitated diffusion of small solute molecules (e.g. glucose and amino acids) are often present in cell membranes. Where transport is in the same direction as the concentration gradient for the solute molecule, facilitated diffusion occurs (e.g. glucose uptake into adipose tissue, brain, liver and skeletal muscle). Rapid metabolism of glucose in the cell prevents slowing of uptake. Stimulation of glucose uptake by insulin in tissues such as adipose tissue and skeletal muscle occurs by the recruitment of glucose transporters, stored in vesicles, to the plasma membrane.

In both the intestine and kidney, solute molecules are actively transported coupled to Na^+ movement (Fig. 3.12.3). In red blood cells, anion exchange contributes both to transport of O_2 and CO_2 and to buffering in the circulation (Fig. 3.12.4).

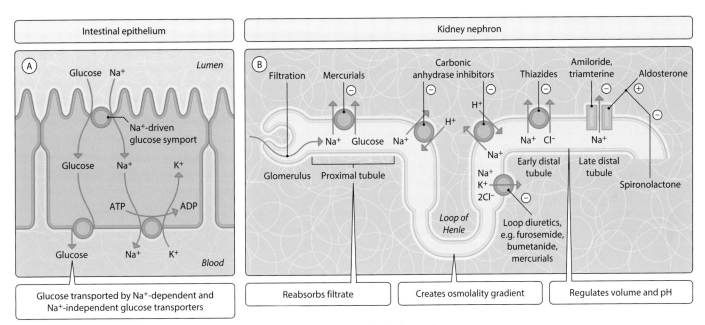

Fig. 3.12.3 Glucose uptake in the gut (A), and sodium reabsorption in the kidney (B).

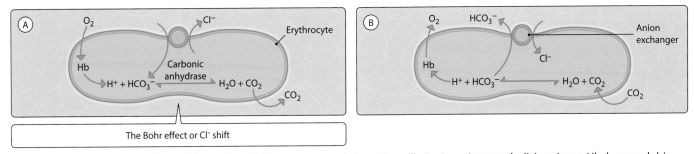

Fig. 3.12.4 Anion exchange in red blood cells. (A) Pulmonary capillaries; (B) capillaries in active metabolizing tissue. Hb, haemoglobin.

13. Protein targeting to different cellular destinations

Questions
- How are proteins targeted to different cellular destinations?
- What is the signal for proteins to enter the secretory pathway?
- How are proteins destined for the endoplasmic reticulum prevented from being secreted?

Proteins are targeted to cellular destinations by specific structural signals within the protein or, in the absence of a specific signal, to a default destination. A complex series of primary and/or secondary structural protein motifs together with appropriate receptor proteins in the target organelle play major roles. Compartment-specific retention signals are also important so that protein activities localized to particular compartments are not randomized during interorganelle vesicular transport.

Secretory pathways
Nascent polypeptides from the rough ER pass initially to the Golgi apparatus (Fig. 3.13.1). Some proteins are arrested by specific targeting signals that locate the protein within the secretory pathway (e.g. protein disulphide isomerase to the ER, glycosyl transferases to the Golgi) (Fig. 3.13.2). A C-terminal amino acid sequence, KDEL, signals retention of the protein in the ER (Fig. 3.13.2). Those proteins that are not sequestered in this way—targeted to other organelles, the plasma membrane or secretion—are sorted in the trans-Golgi network. Proteins may enter either a constitutive or a regulated secretory pathway.

Constitutive pathway
In the constitutive pathway, non-clathrin-coated vesicles bud-off continuously from the trans-Golgi network and migrate to the cytoplasmic face of the plasma membrane. Fusion of the vesicle with the plasma membrane releases secreted proteins and introduces transmembrane proteins into the membrane. Extracellular matrix proteins and protein components of the plasma membrane use the constitutive pathway and it may be that the constitutive pathway is the default pathway for any protein that

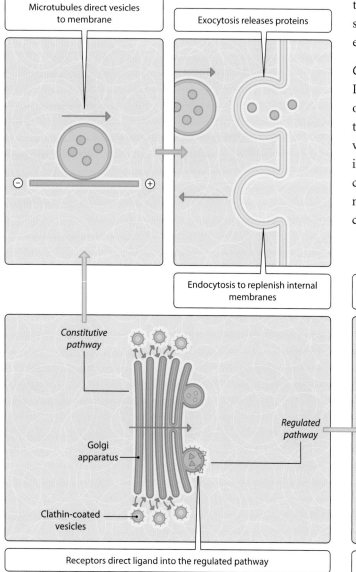

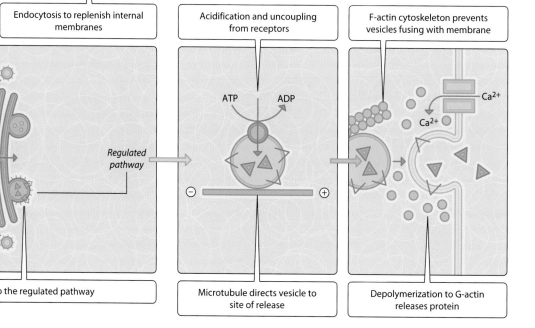

Fig. 3.13.1 Secretory pathways.

does not carry a specific address. The constitutive pathway is Ca^{2+} dependent. The Ca^{2+} may be required for vesicle migration and/or vesicle/membrane fusion. Retrograde vesicular transport replenishes the ER bilayer.

Regulated pathway

Proteins entering the regulated secretory pathway do so at a much higher concentration and are more actively sequestered by binding to aggregated intralumenal receptors in the trans-Golgi network. For example, proinsulin is sequestered by a receptor protein in the trans-Golgi network. The budding-off of vesicles is driven by the formation of a clathrin coat and vesicles are then transferred towards the site of release along microtubular fibres. Near the plasma membrane, the vesicles in the regulated pathway interact with a network of F-actin–fodrin filaments, which hold most of the vesicles away from the membrane, preventing fusion. A local rise in $[Ca^{2+}]_i$, in response to raised glucose concentration, triggers membrane fusion by promoting depolymerization of the F-actin–fodrin matrix, activation of the F-actin-cleaving enzyme gelosin and the capping of actin filaments (p. 68). In nerve terminals, there is evidence that some secretory vesicles in regulated pathways may be linked directly to voltage-gated Ca^{2+} channels by proteins such as synaptotagmin, such that the vesicle is ideally placed for membrane fusion when the local $[Ca^{2+}]$ rises.

Lysosomal targeting via mannose 6-phosphate residues

Rather than receive a complex oligosaccharide modification, the high mannose cores of oligosaccharide chains on enzymes targeted to a lysosomal localization are phosphorylated in the cis-Golgi to mannose 6-phosphate (see Fig. 3.3.3). Phosphorylated mannose serves as the signal for lysosomal targeting by binding to a mannose 6-phosphate receptor (at neutral pH) in the trans-Golgi, which directs the proteins to acidic sorting vesicles (CURL; Ch. 16). The acidic pH releases the enzymes into the lumen, allowing the receptor to recycle to the Golgi apparatus; vesicles containing the lysosomal enzymes can then be directed to their lysosomal destination. In the lysosomal storage diseases (Ch. 3), the inability to digest certain substrates causes the lysosomes to swell. This leads to a wide range of dysfunctions in different tissues and to varying phenotypes.

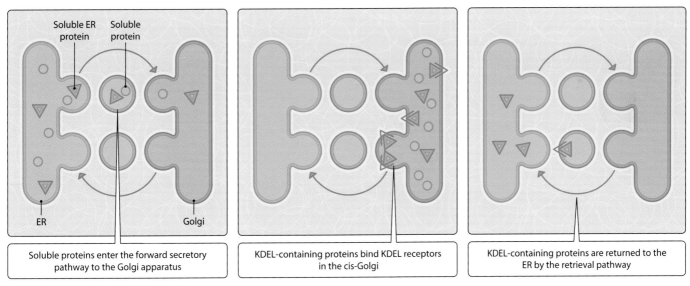

| Soluble proteins enter the forward secretory pathway to the Golgi apparatus | KDEL-containing proteins bind KDEL receptors in the cis-Golgi | KDEL-containing proteins are returned to the ER by the retrieval pathway |

Fig. 3.13.2 Retention of protein in the endoplasmic reticulum (ER).

14. Protein transport into mitochondria and nuclei

Questions
- How do proteins enter mitochondria after translation?
- How is the transfer of large proteins from the cytoplasm to the nucleoplasm and vice versa achieved?
- How does the small G-protein Ran ensure directional transport into and out of the nucleus?

Protein incorporation into mitochondria

Nearly all mitochondrial proteins are synthesized in the cytoplasm and taken up into the mitochondrion post-translationally. Proteins are targeted to mitochondria by short targeting signals, which may be located at the N-terminal or internally within the polypeptide chain. Receptors in the outer mitochondrial membrane recognize the signal and direct the proteins to the import machinery (Fig. 3.14.1). The protein must be unfolded to allow the vectorial translocation across the membrane through the general import pore (GIP) of the translocase of the outer membrane (TOM) complex. Cytosolic chaperone proteins stabilize the unfolded proteins before translocation commences. After crossing the outer membrane, imported preproteins are directed to different translocase of the inner membrane (TIM) complexes depending on the nature of the signal sequence (Fig. 3.14.1). Those proteins with N-terminal preprotein signals are translocated through the TIM23 complex,

driven by the membrane potential, an ATP-dependent motor and chaperone proteins (heat shock protein (hsp) 70), which stabilize the unfolded proteins as they are translocated. Once in the matrix, the N-terminal mitochondrial signal sequence is cleaved by the mitochondrial processing peptidase (MPP) and the transported protein folds into its mature structure assisted by the chaperone protein hsp60. Some preproteins contain internal hydrophobic membrane-spanning domains that act as stop-transfer sequences in the inner membrane or act to assist protein insertion from the matrix. Some other proteins, with an internal signal sequence, destined for the inner membrane enter a separate TIM pathway involving the TIM22 complex. This pathway relies on the mitochondrial membrane potential and a family of small TIM chaperone proteins to facilitate transfer of the protein through the intermembrane space.

Nuclear pores in protein transport

Selective nuclear pore structures punctuate the nuclear envelope and allow the uninhibited two-way passage of small molecules and proteins up to ~ 60 kDa. They also provide the exit route for newly formed mRNA and ribosome complexes and a selective receptor-mediated mechanism for the ATP-hydrolysis-dependent import of larger proteins (> 90 kDa) bearing appropriate targeting signal motifs. Several short primary sequences that target proteins to the nucleus have been

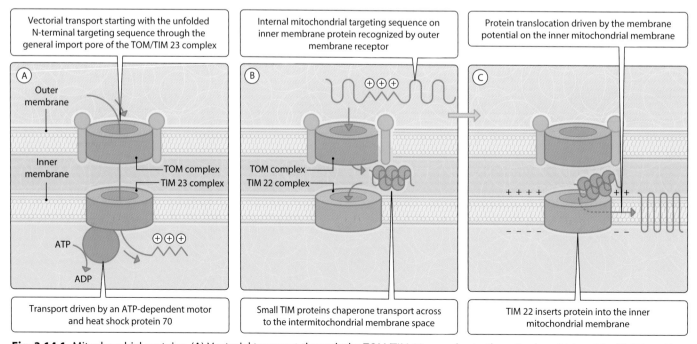

Fig. 3.14.1 Mitochondrial proteins. (A) Vectorial transport through the TOM/TIM 23 complex to the mitochondrial matrix; (B,C) insertion of proteins into the inner mitochondrial membrane by the TOM/TIM 22 complex.

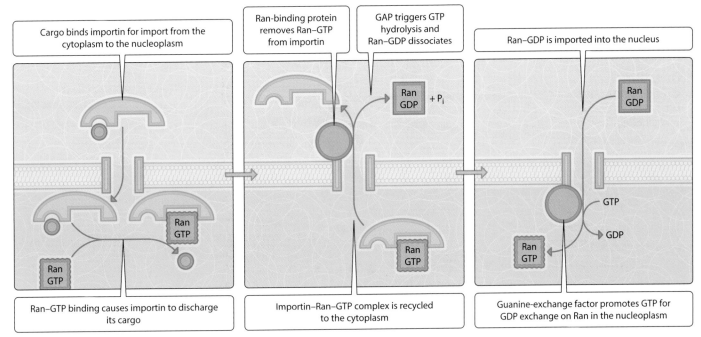

Fig. 3.14.2 Role of importins and Ran in the transport of proteins into the nucleus.

identified. A family of nuclear import receptor proteins, **importins**, for different signals is involved in recognition (Fig. 3.14.2). On complex formation, the importins interact with filamentous nucleoporin, which guides ATP-driven movement into the nuclear pore.

The small G-protein GTPase **Ran**, which may exist in two conformations depending on whether GDP or GTP is bound, drives directional transport through nuclear pores. On entry of the importin–nuclear protein complex into the nucleoplasm, Ran-GTP binds to importin causing it to discharge its nuclear-

targeted cargo. The empty importin–Ran-GTP complex is cycled back to the cytoplasm, where Ran-binding protein strips off the bound Ran-GTP. GTPase-activating protein (GAP) then acts to trigger GTP hydrolysis. Ran-GDP dissociates from the Ran-binding protein and is imported back into the nucleus where guanine-exchange factor (GEF) promotes the replacement of GDP with GTP, converting Ran-GDP to Ran-GTP to complete the cycle. In contrast, binding of nuclear proteins to nuclear export receptors, **exportins**, is augmented in the presence of Ran-GTP (Fig. 3.14.3).

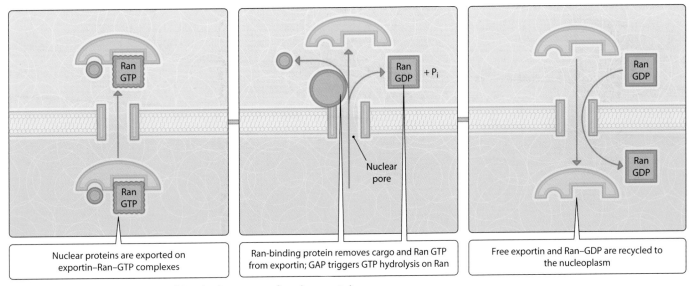

Fig. 3.14.3 Role of exportins and Ran in the export of nuclear proteins.

15. Membrane vesicle transport

Questions
- How does the uptake of particulates and solutes differ?
- What is the driving force for transport vesicle formation?
- What is the function of SNAREs in vesicular transport?

Phagocytosis and pinocytosis

Phagocytosis is the internalization of receptor-bound particulate material by the evagination of psuedopods and a membrane 'zippering-mechanism' to engulf the particle for degradation in lysosomes. In mammals, this process is found only in specialized cells (e.g. macrophages and neutrophils). Pinocytosis, leading to the uptake of solutes and retrieval of plasma membrane to balance that inserted by the secretory pathways, occurs by membrane invagination. 'Fluid-phase' endocytosis permits the uptake of entrapped solutes, while receptor-mediated endocytosis provides a mechanism for the selective uptake of molecules bound to cell-surface receptors. Most endocytic vesicles ultimately fuse with primary lysosomes to form secondary lysosomes, in which internalized materials are digested.

Membrane trafficking

Trafficking between membrane-bounded organelles is mediated by small membrane vesicles, which bud and pinch-off from the source organelle and bind and fuse with the target organelle. Assembly of coat proteins into basket-like structures drives vesicle formation and sequesters appropriate membrane proteins.

Different coat proteins (e.g. clathrin, COPI and COPII and caveolin) are involved in different transport steps in the cell; for example, COPI buds vesicles from the ER and COPII buds vesicles from the Golgi cisternae. Passage between organelles is directed along microtubule cytoskeletal elements in an ATP-dependent process (Ch. 38) before vesicles are uncoated to permit fusion with the target vesicle.

Coat formation is initiated by specific guanine-nucleotide exchange factors (GEFs) in the membrane binding to cytosolic coat-recruitment GTPases. The GDP bound to the inactive state is released, allowing GTP to bind and activate a conformational change in the protein. A covalently linked fatty acid moiety is 'unmasked'; this inserts into the membrane and recruits coat proteins to begin coat assembly. Slow hydrolysis of GTP by the coat-recruitment GTPases reforms the resting conformation and withdraws the fatty acid tail from the membrane.

Targeting of transport vesicles by SNARE proteins

The SNARE hypothesis proposes that each transport vesicle possesses one or more specific SNARE proteins (vSNARE) in its membrane and that this protein binds to cognate SNAREs in the target membrane (tSNARE), thereby ensuring correct targeting of the vesicle (Fig. 3.15.1). Soluble NSF (*N*-ethylmaleimide-sensitive fusion proteins) attachment proteins (SNAPs) are thought to bind to interacting SNAREs (SNAP receptors), which, in turn, permit the binding of NSF proteins to complete the docking and fusion particle. The intertwining of the interacting SNAREs drives out water from between the fusing membranes and facilitates membrane fusion.

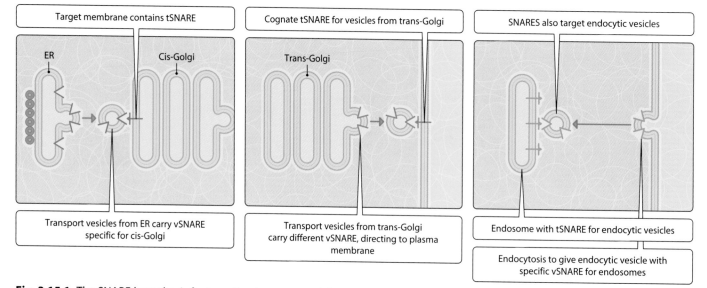

Fig. 3.15.1 The SNARE hypothesis for targeting transport vesicles.

Vesicle docking

Like coat formation, vesicle docking is mediated by monomeric GTPases of the Rab family (Fig. 3.15.2). It is proposed that GEF.V activation of exchange of GTP for GDP results in a conformational change that exposes a lipid tail anchor that targets the donor organelle. The Rab-GTP in the transport vesicle docks with a Rab effector in the target organelle and facilitates intereaction of the appropriate v- and tSNARE pairs. On hydrolysis of GTP, Rab-GDP re-enters the cytoplasm.

 DISEASES OF MEMBRANE VESICULAR TRANSPORT

Alterations to proteins involved in vesicle recognition and membrane fusion are increasingly implicated in human disease. For example, loss of function of Rab GTPases is associated with immune impairment, bleeding, mental retardation and kidney disease, while overexpression of Rab has been associated with cardiac hypertrophy, thyroid disease and a variety of cancers. (See also lysosomal storage disease; Ch. 3.)

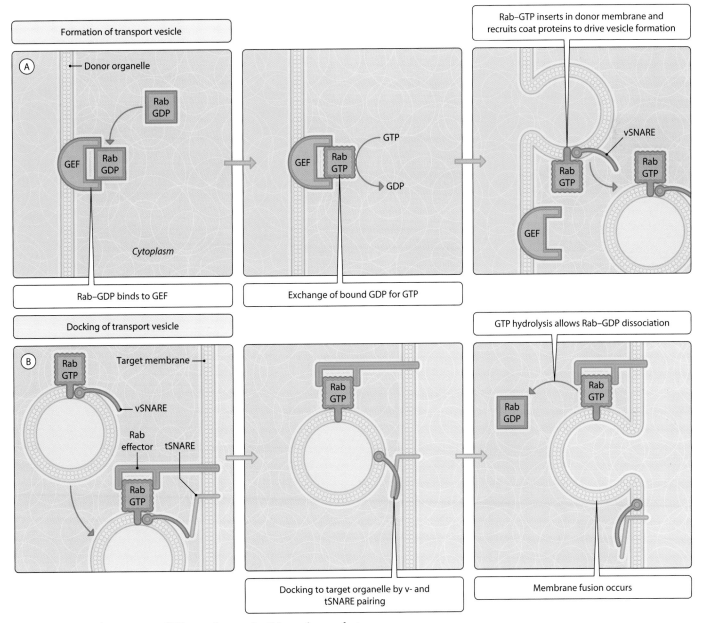

Fig. 3.15.2 Vesicle transport. GEF, guanine-nucleotide-exchange factor.

16. Receptor-mediated endocytosis

Questions
- How is the uncoating of coated vesicles and the uncoupling of receptor and ligand achieved?
- How do cells use receptor-mediated endocytosis?
- How may viruses take advantage of this process?

Uptake of cholesterol: an example of receptor-mediated endocytosis

Cholesterol is carried in the circulation in large spherical particles that originate in the liver, called low density lipoproteins (LDLs). Each LDL contains a non-polar core of cholesterol molecules esterified to long-chain fatty acids, surrounded by a lipid layer containing phospholipids, cholesterol and a single protein species, apoprotein B.

Cells that require cholesterol synthesize cell surface receptors (LDL receptor) that recognize apoprotein B specifically (Fig. 3.16.1). Within 10 min of binding, the LDL particle is internalized and delivered to the lysosomes, where the cholesterol is released from the cholesterol esters. LDL receptors are localized in clusters over small indentations or pits with a bristle-like appearance, termed **coated pits**. The coated pits invaginate and pinch-off constitutively from the plasma membrane to form coated vesicles, resulting in the internalization of receptors whether or not they are occupied by

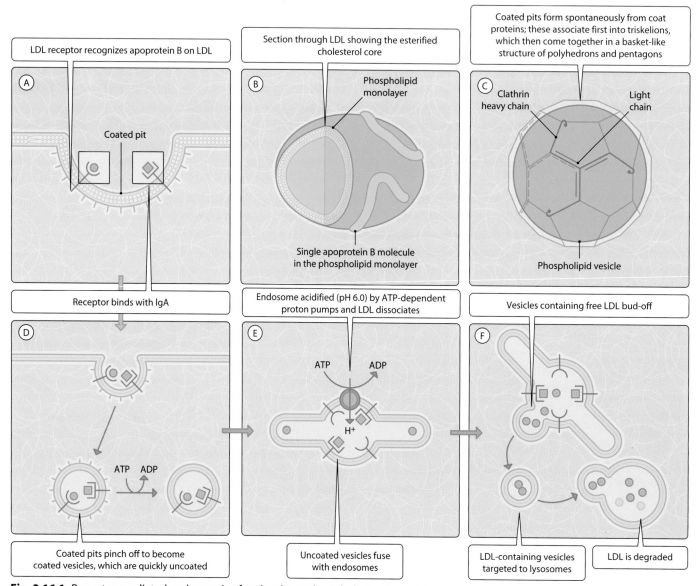

Fig. 3.16.1 Receptor-mediated endocytosis of molecules such as cholesterol and IgA.

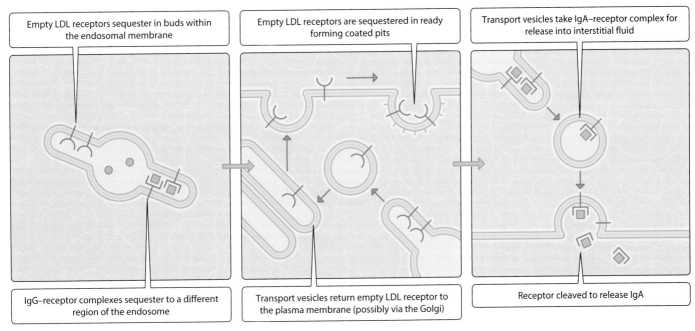

Fig. 3.16.2 Return of receptors to coated pits.

ligand. The association of the coat protein clathrin is energy independent and, therefore, coated-pit formation is spontaneous. Coated vesicles are quickly uncoated by an ATP-dependent uncoating protein, which binds and stabilizes the freed coat proteins; the uncoated vesicles then fuse with larger smooth vesicles called endosomes. The pH of the endosome is maintained between approximately 5.5 and 6.0 by an ATP-dependent proton pump (Fig. 3.16.1). At this pH, the LDL receptor has a low affinity for the LDL particle and the two dissociate. The endosome is also known as the 'compartment for the uncoupling of receptor and ligand' (CURL). The transmembranous receptors are sequestered and bud-off in vesicles to be recycled to the plasma membrane. Recycled receptors are inserted randomly in the plasma membrane but are quickly sequestered again into coated pits (Fig. 3.16.2). The contents of the endosome are passed on to lysosomes where the cholesterol is deesterified and released into the cell. Whether this involves fusion of endosomes and lysosomes or the passage of transport vesicles between compartments remains to be resolved. Thus, the LDLs and their receptors are sorted from each other in the endosome.

Modes of receptor-mediated endocytosis

Receptors for different ligands enter the cell via the same coated pits and the pathway from coated pits to the endosome is common for all proteins that undergo endocytosis. Different modes of this process can be defined on the basis of the destination of internalized receptor and ligand. Receptors targeted to different cellular destinations, by short amino acid motifs, are sorted within the CURL to discrete regions of membrane, which bud-off into transport vesicles.

Mode 1. The ligand is degraded and the receptor recycled (e.g. LDL uptake).

Mode 2. The ligand and the receptor are recycled (e.g. transferrin with two ferric ions (Fe^{3+}) bound is internalized bound to the transferrin receptor). In the CURL, the Fe^{3+} is released by the acidic environment but the apotransferrin (without Fe^{3+} bound) remains bound to the receptor and is recycled back to the plasma membrane, where, at pH 7.4, the apotransferrin dissociates from the transferrin receptor again.

Mode 3. The ligand and the receptor are degraded. For example, insulin receptors may be downregulated by receptor-mediated endocytosis, resulting in desensitization of the cell. Insulin remains bound to its receptor in the CURL and both are targeted to the lysosomes for degradation.

Mode 4. Transcytosis occurs. For example, maternal immunoglobulins remain bound to their receptors in placenta and are transported across the cell to the fetal circulation. Immunoglobulin is released by proteolysis of the receptor, resulting in a bound 'secretory component' derived from the receptor.

VIRUSES AND TOXINS

Membrane-enveloped viruses and some toxins exploit endocytic pathways to enter cells after binding to receptors in the plasma membrane. Once in the endosome, where the acid pH is favourable, the viral membrane is able to fuse with the endosomal membrane, thereby releasing the viral RNA into the cell where it can be translated and replicated to form new viral particles.

17. The resting membrane potential

Questions
- How do cells maintain the resting membrane potential?
- What are the relative contributions of Na⁺/K⁺-ATPase and voltage-insensitive K⁺ channels in setting membrane potential?
- How do cells change the resting membrane potential?

Membrane potential

All cells have an electrical potential difference across their plasma membrane (membrane potential). This is always expressed as the voltage inside relative to that outside the cell. Animal cells have resting membrane potentials ranging from approximately −20 to −90 mV depending on the cell type (Fig. 3.17.1). Changes in this potential difference form the basis of electrical signalling in cells.

The resting membrane potential

At rest, cell membranes are more permeable to K⁺ than to other ionic species because of facilitated diffusion through K⁺ channel proteins, which form K⁺-specific pores in the membrane. The extracellular and intracellular K⁺ concentrations in a 'typical' cell are 4.5 and 160 mmol/l, respectively; therefore, K⁺ tends to move outwards down its concentration gradient. Since large protein anions inside the cell are unable to follow K⁺ out of the cell, a negative potential develops on the intracellular face of the plasma membrane. This growing potential difference then opposes the further efflux of K⁺. An equilibrium is reached when the diffusional and electrical forces are balanced and there is no net movement of K⁺. At equilibrium, the potential across the membrane is termed the potassium equilibrium potential (E_K).

Although the passage of K⁺ through K⁺ channels predominates in the resting cell, the resting membrane potential never reaches E_K. This is because the plasma membrane is not totally impermeable to other ions and the passage of these ions through selective ion channels contributes to the overall membrane potential. Note that very few ions need to move across the plasma membrane to establish a membrane potential.

Proteins involved in setting membrane potential

The activity of Na⁺/K⁺-ATPase provides the outward ionic gradient for K⁺ necessary for maintenance of the membrane potential. Although electrogenic (three Na⁺ outwards for two K⁺ inwards in each reaction cycle), this enzyme contributes little to resting membrane potential (approximately −5 mV). Voltage-insensitive K⁺ channels, which remain open despite changes in potential across the membrane, are responsible predominantly for the K⁺ movement that establishes the resting membrane potential. These channels contain a pore-forming structure (S5–S6) similar to that in voltage-sensitive K⁺ channels but lack a voltage sensor (S1–S4) (Ch. 19).

Changing the membrane potential

Changing the permeability of the plasma membrane to a particular ion causes a change in membrane potential towards the equilibrium potential for that ion (Fig. 3.17.2). Thus, opening K⁺

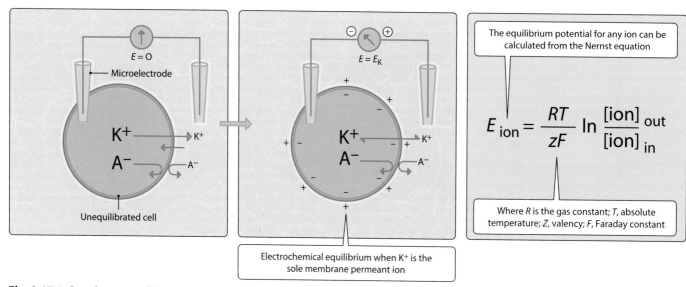

$$E_{ion} = \frac{RT}{zF} \ln \frac{[ion]_{out}}{[ion]_{in}}$$

The equilibrium potential for any ion can be calculated from the Nernst equation

Where R is the gas constant; T, absolute temperature; Z, valency; F, Faraday constant

E = 0   Microelectrode   Unequilibrated cell

E = E_K Electrochemical equilibrium when K⁺ is the sole membrane permeant ion

Fig. 3.17.1 Development of the resting membrane potential.

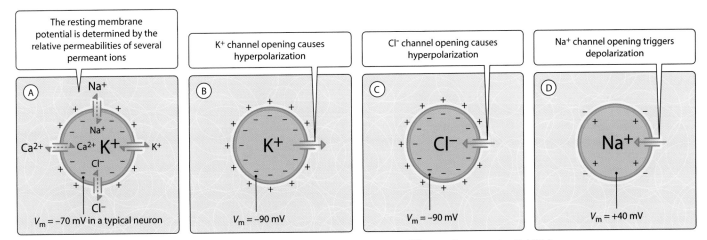

Fig. 3.17.2 Increasing the membrane permeability for a particular ion can modify membrane potential (V_m).

or Cl⁻ channels results in the inside of the cell becoming more negative. This is termed **hyperpolarization**. Conversely, opening Na⁺ or Ca²⁺ channels results in the inside of the cell becoming less negative. This is termed **depolarization**. Channels can exist in three major states: open, closed or inactivated. Alterations in the opening or closing of different ion channels via their gating mechanisms allow the membrane potential of the cell to be changed. Channel gating occurs by two main mechanisms:

- ligand-gating, where binding of a ligand to a receptor site on the channel results in channel opening (or closing); the ligand may be an extracellular signalling molecule or an intracellular messenger, depending on the channel type (Ch. 22)
- voltage-gating, where the channel opens or closes in response to changes in the membrane potential.

INCREASED MEMBRANE EXCITABILITY IN HYPERKALAEMIA

The consequences of hyperkalaemia (raised extracellular K⁺ concentration) are a less-negative E_K and, hence, a less-negative resting membrane potential (Fig. 3.17.3). Cellular electrical activity depends on the ability to depolarize membranes (see below). Therefore, in acute hyperkalaemia, a lesser change in ion conductance is required to depolarize the heart and so excite cardiac membranes, resulting in ventricular arrhythmia, which can be life threatening. After electrical activity, Na⁺ channels become inactivated (Ch. 18). In chronic hyperkalaemia, a less-negative membrane potential also prevents the repriming of inactivated Na⁺ channels, resulting in an electrically silent or 'accommodated' membrane; this also contributes to the arrhythmia.

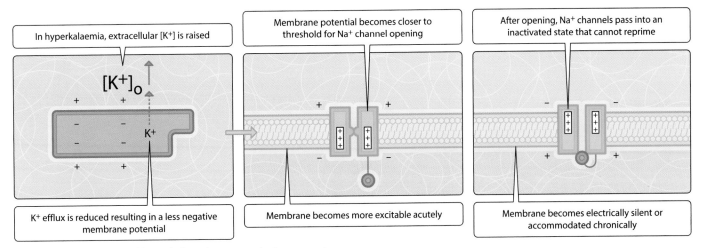

Fig. 3.17.3 The effect of hyperkalaemia on ventricular myocytes.

18. Electrical signalling: the action potential

Questions
- What is the molecular basis of the action potential in nerve fibres?
- Nerve fibres become refractory to further action potentials just after the firing of an action potential. Why does this occur?
- How are action potentials initiated?

The action potential

Electrical signals are propagated over the plasma membrane of electrically excitable cells by electrical events called action potentials. During the action potential, the membrane depolarizes briefly before repolarizing to the resting condition (Fig. 3.18.1). The depolarizing phase of the action potential is generated by an increase in membrane permeability to Na^+

through the opening of voltage-gated Na^+ channels. The flow of Na^+ inwards, down its electrochemical gradient, drives the membrane potential towards the equilibrium potential for Na^+ (E_{Na}), thereby depolarizing the membrane. Soon after activation, Na^+ channels pass from an open to an inactivated conformation, reducing the rate of Na^+ influx back to resting levels

In addition to the inactivation of Na^+ channels, in most cells voltage-gated K^+ channels with slower activation kinetics than Na^+ channels (delayed rectifier channels: K_{DR} channels) open. The resulting efflux of K^+ down its electrochemical gradient results in the repolarization of the membrane; in some cells (e.g. in nerve axons), the membrane potential can hyperpolarize to a value more negative than the original resting potential before returning once again to the resting membrane potential on inactivation of the K^+ channels.

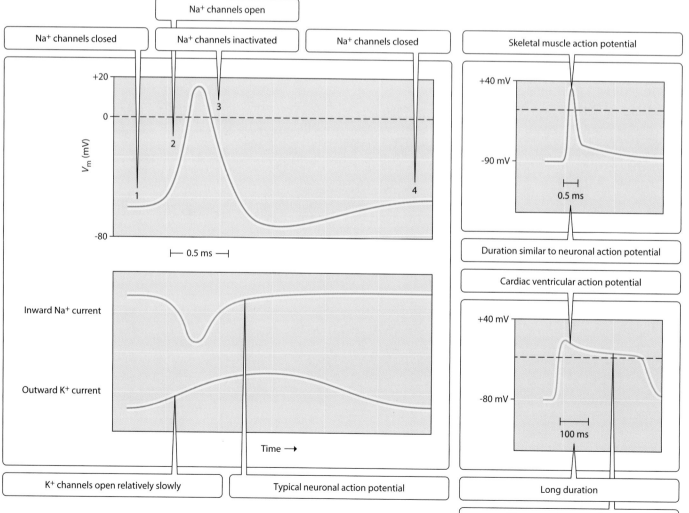

Fig. 3.18.1 The action potential.

The duration of an action potential in nerve axon and skeletal muscle is approximately 0.5–1.0 ms. Longer-duration action potentials ($\approx$ 100 ms) are seen in cardiac ventricular muscle owing to the opening of Ca^{2+} channels with relatively slow activation and inactivation kinetics and closure of inward rectifier K^+ channels.

Initiation of an action potential

Initiation of an action potential depends on the membrane potential rising above a threshold value (approximately −50 mV). This may occur either through (a) an increased open probability (P_o) for voltage-gated Na^+ or Ca^{2+} channels, which leads to membrane depolarization to exceed the hyperpolarizing effect of the resting K^+ efflux or (b) the closure of K^+ channels, which reduces the hyperpolarizing influence on the membrane, allowing the membrane potential to rise through the leak of Na^+ and Ca^{2+}. Because there is a threshold for initiation, action potentials are all or nothing. The progress of a wave of depolarization over a cell membrane is then caused by the self-reinforcing way in which Na^+ channels open: that is, the depolarizing phase of an action potential at one point on the cell membrane, by local current flow, will raise the membrane potential in adjacent regions of the membrane sufficiently to exceed the threshold for action potential initiation in that region (Ch. 20).

Inactivation of voltage-gated cation channels

Voltage-gated channels pass through three states from closed, through open, to an inactivated state on depolarization. Once in the inactivated state, a channel cannot reopen until it has been 're-primed' by repolarization of the membrane (Fig. 3.18.2). Consequently, once inactivated, Na^+ channels cannot be reopened during an action potential. This property is important because it prevents irreversible depolarization of the membrane, permits directionality to nerve impulse conduction and also allows information to be coded with respect to the frequency at which action potentials are fired. Directly after the onset of an action potential, there is an 'absolute refractory period', during which the membrane cannot be further excited, followed by a 'relative refractory period', during which it becomes progressively easier to elicit a further action potential as the Na^+ channels recover from inactivation.

ANTIARRHYTHMIC DRUGS

Antiarrhythmic drugs alter heart rate by indirectly or directly blocking ion fluxes across the myocyte membranes. Change in heart rate may be achieved by prolonging the refractory period (Na^+ and K^+ channel blockers), reducing sympathetic stimulation (beta-blockers) or reducing conduction at the sinoatrial and atrioventricular nodes (L-type Ca^{2+} channel blockers).

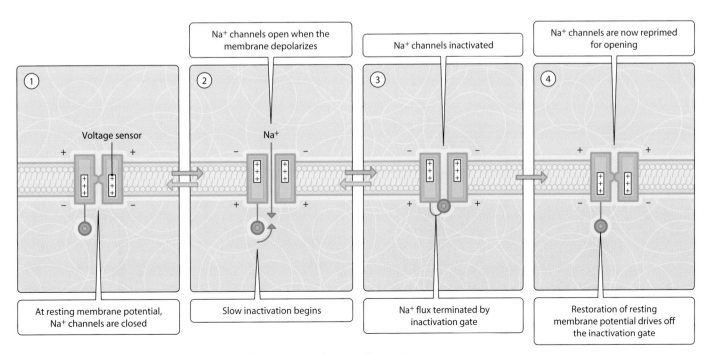

Fig. 3.18.2 Action, inactivation and priming of voltage-gated cation channels.

19. Ion channels

Questions
- How is opening of membrane ion channels gated by changes in membrane potential?
- What is the molecular basis of closed, open and inactivated states in voltage-gated ion channels?
- How do ion channels contribute to channelopathies?

Voltage-gated cation channels
Voltage-gated (also known as voltage-operated or voltage-sensitive) cation channels share a common basic design based on a core structure of six hydrophobic membrane-spanning segments (S1–S6) (Fig. 3.19.1). The loop-linking segments S5 and S6 (H5) folds back into the membrane as a hairpin loop to form the pore lining. Four structural units are required to constitute a channel pore. Voltage sensitivity is conferred by the S4 transmembrane segment (voltage sensor), which contains a positively charged residue (lysine or arginine) at every third position in the primary sequence. The outward movement of this segment in response to the electrical force imposed by membrane depolarization is thought to drive the opening of voltage-gated channels. In those voltage-gated channels that inactivate rapidly, an inactivation 'ball' swings into a vestibule 'ball acceptor' domain on channel activation to block the pore. This ball is derived from the N-terminal region in these K+ channels (N-type inactivation). A second relatively rapid form of inactivation (C-type) has been characterized in some K+ channels. In Na+ and Ca2+ channels, which comprise four linked repeating channel units, cytoplasmic loops rather than the N-terminal domain form the ball.

Anion channels
A family of anion-selective channels (CLC) that conduct Cl− predominantly have important functions in cell volume regulation, NaCl movement in kidney tubules and a background hyperpolarizing Cl− current in skeletal muscle.

Auxiliary subunits of channels
Pore-forming polypeptides often coassemble with accessory subunits. Accessory subunits can play important roles in determining the kinetic properties of the channel and in targeting and anchoring of the channel (Fig. 3.19.2).

Channel modulation
Channel activity may be modulated in response to activation of parallel signalling pathways to integrate signalling responses. Often this occurs by channel phosphorylation/ dephosphorylation mechanisms following activation of protein kinases or phosphatases. Modulation may also occur by the direct interaction of G-protein subunits or of cellular metabolites such as Ca2+, free fatty acids and nitric oxide.

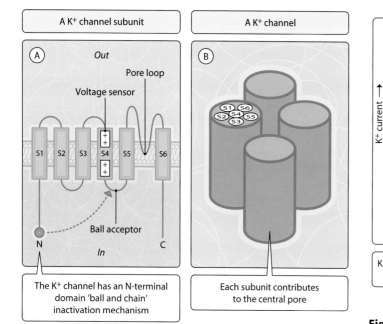

Fig. 3.19.1 Voltage-gated cation channels.

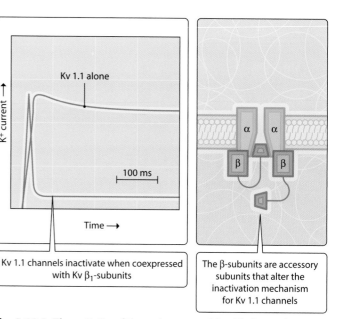

Fig. 3.19.2 The activity of the voltage-sensitive K+ channel Kv1.1 is altered by expression with the Kvβ₁-subunit.

CHANNELOPATHIES

Channelopathies are disorders caused by pathology of ion channel function and usually are clinically characterized by episodes of disturbed excitability of nerve or muscle cells. These diseases are usually caused by mutations in genes encoding ion channels inducing changes in channel gating.

Channel mutations in myotonia

Several forms of myotonia (muscle stiffness owing to increased muscle excitability and contractility) have been associated with point mutations in genes for Na^+ channels (Fig. 3.19.3). Many of these mutations result in slowed inactivation of the channel and, therefore, prolonged excitation of the muscle membrane. Point mutations in the skeletal muscle Cl^- channel isoform CLC-1 that reduce Cl^- conductance and, thereby, increase muscle excitability have been characterized in patients with inherited myotonias such as myotonia congenita (Thomsen's disease) and generalized myotonia (Becker's myotonia).

Channel mutations in long QT syndrome

Long QT syndrome is a group of inherited cardiac arrhythmias in which repolarization of the ventricle is delayed, resulting in a prolonged QT interval in the electrocardiogram. Genetic analysis has revealed mutations in a variety of channels that may be responsible. Mutations affecting the Na^+ channel cause long QT syndrome, slow inactivation and result in prolongation of the cardiac action potential. In contrast, mutations in LCNQ1, minK or HERG K^+ channel subunits often cause a dominant negative reduction in components of the K^+ current that normally repolarizes the cardiac membrane at the end of the action potential.

Renal epithelial Na^+ channels and hypertension

In Liddle's disease, mutations affecting the renal epithelial Na^+ channel cause excessive Na^+ reabsorbtion from kidney tubules and increased water retention, resulting in increased blood pressure. Similarly, hypertension resulting from raised aldosterone levels in the rare syndromes of glucocorticoid-remediable aldosteronism and apparent mineralocorticoid excess is a consequence of increased activity of renal epithelial Na^+ channels.

Cystic fibrosis transmembrane conductance regulator

The epithelial cell cystic fibrosis transmembrane conductance regulator (CFTR) Cl^- conducting channel opens in response to phosphorylation by cyclic AMP-dependent protein kinase. The Cl^- efflux from epithelia is followed by water movement. In cystic fibrosis, point mutations in the *CFTR* gene result in defective Cl^- transport and reduced outward water movement, leading to secretion of abnormally thick mucus. In the lung, this can lead to difficulty in breathing and at other sites this abnormality leads to inflammatory responses, infection and progressive damage, which contribute to the development of the disease.

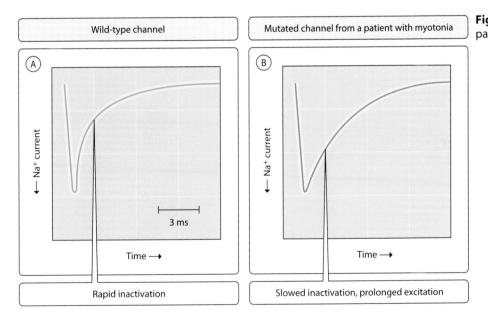

Fig. 3.19.3 Effect of mutations on current passed by Na^+ channels.

20. Electrical conduction in nerves

Questions
- How are electrical impulses carried in a nerve cell?
- How is re-entrant excitation prevented in a region of nerve that has just fired an action potential?
- What factors govern the conduction velocity of nerves?
- What is saltatory conduction in nerve fibres? Why does it occur? How does saltatory conduction influence conduction velocity in nerve fibres?

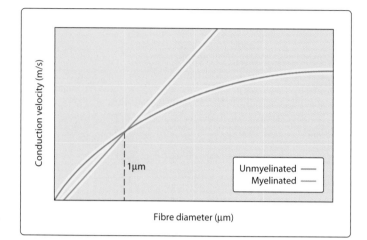

Fig. 3.20.2 Relationship between conduction velocity and nerve fibre diameter.

Impulse propagation

Nerve impulses propagate via local currents that are induced within the nerve after firing of an action potential. During an action potential, the active region of membrane becomes more positively charged inside compared with adjacent regions and more negative outside compared with adjacent regions. Induced local currents raise adjacent resting regions of the nerve membrane to threshold for firing of an action potential, thereby propagating the electrical signal along the nerve membrane (Fig. 3.20.1).

The conduction velocity of an action potential over the surface of a nerve cell depends on the size of the cell and the electrical capacity of the cell membrane. The internal (axoplasmic) electrical resistance to local current flow is larger in nerve fibres of smaller diameter. Thus, conduction velocity is faster in larger nerve fibres (Fig. 3.20.2). Conduction velocity is also related to the electrical capacity of the cell membrane (i.e. the ability to

store electric charge). A low membrane capacitance results in increased conduction velocity as less work is required to depolarize adjacent regions of membrane to threshold for an action potential to be fired. In other words, conduction velocity is faster when the electrical resistance of the membrane is high.

Conduction of electrical signals is directional

After an action potential has fired in a region of nerve membrane, that part of the membrane becomes refractory to the firing of a second action potential because of the inactivation of

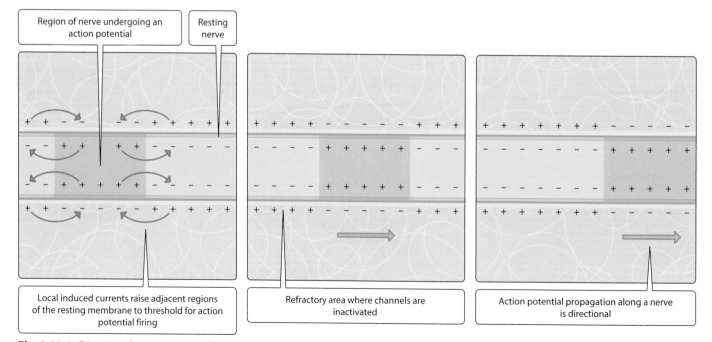

Fig. 3.20.1 Directional propagating of an action potential in a nerve.

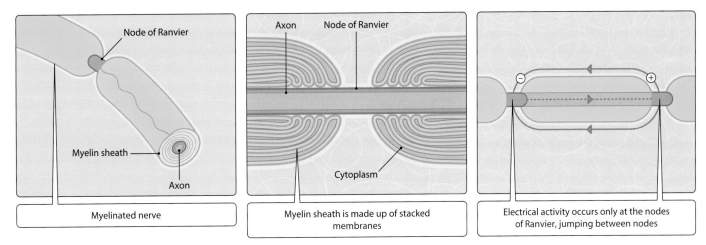

Fig. 3.20.3 Nerve conduction in myelinated nerves.

Na$^+$ channels. Therefore, a nerve impulse cannot re-enter a region of nerve axon that has just fired. In this way, an electrical signal is propagated directionally down a nerve axon.

Myelination

Myelinated nerves are formed from about 4 months of gestation by glial cells, which form a concentric wrapping of up to 200 layers thick around the nerve fibre to create a myelin sheath (Fig. 3.20.3). The cytoplasmic contents are withdrawn, resulting in a multilayered membrane covering. Two types of glial cell are involved: **oligodendrocytes** in the central nervous system (CNS) and **Schwann cells** on peripheral nerves. The length of nerve wrapped by the myelin sheath of one glial cell (1 mm) is termed the **internode**. The unmyelinated regions between internodes are called **nodes of Ranvier**. Myelination reduces substantially the electrical capacitance of the internodal length such that electrical activity occurs only at the nodes of Ranvier. As a result, nerve impulse conduction occurs in a saltatory (jumping) manner, so increasing conduction velocity (Fig. 3.20.3). In myelinated nerves, the Na$^+$ channels that generate action potentials are located exclusively at the nodes of Ranvier. In some myelinated nerves, repolarization does not involve voltage-gated K$^+$ channels because the resting K$^+$ permeability is sufficient to restore the negative resting membrane potential.

If demyelination occurs, the excitation of successive nodes becomes progressively slowed because of the increased membrane capacitance, which causes local current dissipation, and conduction of the action potential ultimately fails. Insertion of new Na$^+$ channels in internodal regions of the membrane can restore some excitability after complete demyelination but conduction velocity in this case is slowed.

Cellular response to action potentials

In addition to propagating the nerve impulse, action potentials may produce a biochemical response in regions of the cell in which they are generated. By stimulating the opening of voltage-gated Ca^{2+} channels, the action potential can produce a rise in free [Ca^{2+}]$_i$, which acts as an intracellular messenger to couple electrical excitation to cellular responses. For example, Ca^{2+} entering presynaptic nerve terminals is a trigger for transmitter release.

MULTIPLE SCLEROSIS

Multiple sclerosis is a disease of demyelination that occurs as a result of autoimmune attack of the myelin sheath around nerves. Symptoms, such as loss of feeling, visual disturbance and muscle weakness, arise from dysfunctional sensory and motor neuron systems where fast axonal transmission is required.

21. Cell-to-cell signalling

Questions
- What is the difference between a hormone, a local mediator and a neurotransmitter?
- What is a ligand?
- What is the difference between a receptor and an acceptor?

Intercellular communication

In multicellular organisms where different functions are carried out by differentiated cells, mechanisms for intercellular communication are required to ensure the efficient integration of cellular activities, or homeostasis. Signalling between cells may occur directly, through gap junctions between cells (Ch. 30) or activation of contact-dependent signalling pathways (Ch. 33), or indirectly, via the secretion of extracellular chemical messengers, which cause a response in a target cell when recognized by specific receptors.

Chemical signalling

Intercellular chemical signals may be classified according to their functions into hormones, local mediators and neurotransmitters (Fig. 3.21.1).

Hormones. These are secreted by specialized cells, usually found in endocrine glands, into the circulation and are carried to target cells where they have their effect. Endocrine signalling coordinates the activities of distally related tissues.

Local mediators. Many cells release local mediators into the extracellular fluid, where they produce responses in cells in the same area of the tissue. These mediators are often short-lived chemical species and are not found generally in the circulation. Signalling by local mediators is referred to as **paracrine** signalling.

Neurotransmitters. Nerve cells release neurotransmitters at nerve terminals into specialized junctions between cells called **synapses**. Diffusion of the neurotransmitter across the synapse and binding to receptors on the postsynaptic membrane permits targeted transfer of information between adjacent cells. A single molecule may fall into more than one of these categories depending on where it is synthesized and released.

Chemical signals

A molecule that binds specifically to a receptor site is termed a ligand. Ligand binding may produce an activation of a receptor. In this case the ligand is termed an **agonist**. Alternatively, a ligand may combine with a receptor site without causing activation. This type of ligand is termed an **antagonist** because it would oppose the action of an agonist. Agonists that stimulate a receptor but are unable to elicit the maximum cell response possible are termed **partial agonists**.

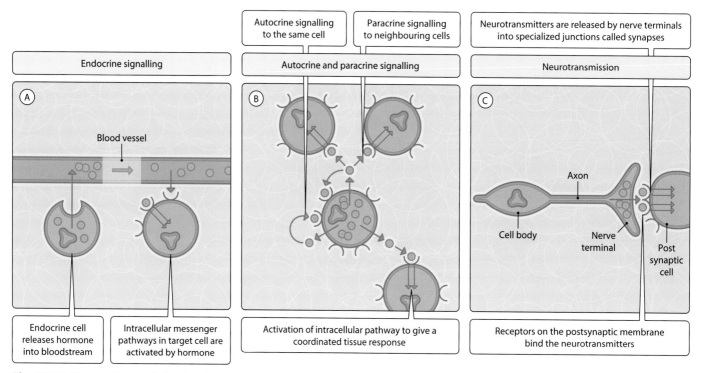

Fig. 3.21.1 Types of intercellular signal.

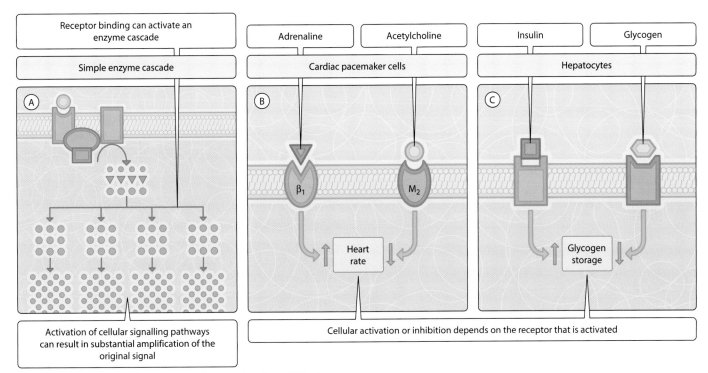

Fig. 3.21.2 Cellular activation or inhibition after ligand binding to a receptor.

Receptors for chemical signals

For a cell to respond to any chemical messenger it must produce specific receptor proteins that recognize and produce a response to the signalling molecule. A receptor is a molecule that recognizes specifically a ligand, or family of ligands, and which in response to ligand binding brings about regulation of a cellular process. In the unbound state, a receptor is functionally silent. Receptors bind ligands with relatively high specificity and affinity (dissociation constants between 10^{-6} and 10^{-9} mol/l; the dissociation constant equals the concentration of ligand necessary to fill 50% of the available receptor sites, c.f. K_M of enzymes).

Acceptors

Many molecules whose activities are modified by the binding of ligands, including drugs, are not strictly receptors under the above definition. If their basic function can be carried out without the interaction of a ligand then they are not, by definition, a receptor. For example, the enzyme dihydrofolate reductase is inhibited by the binding of the antileukaemia drug methotrexate, and it is sometimes referred to as the 'methotrexate receptor'.

This enzyme operates normally in the absence of methotrexate and so is not strictly a receptor but an acceptor.

Amplification of extracellular signals

The concentration of many extracellular signalling molecules is very low (10^{-12}–10^{-6} mol/l). On binding a receptor, signalling molecules activate a cascade of molecular events resulting in considerable amplification of the original signal. This is often achieved by stimulation of enzyme activity (Fig. 3.21.2).

Cellular activation or inhibition

Responses to receptor activation can lead to cellular activation or inhibition depending on the receptor. For example:

- in cardiac pacemaker cells, noradrenaline acting on β_1-adrenoceptors produces an increased heart rate, while acetylcholine acting on M_2 muscarinic receptors produces a slowing of the heart rate
- in hepatocytes, insulin stimulates the synthesis of glycogen from glucose and inhibits glycogen breakdown, while glucagon inhibits glycogen synthesis and stimulates glycogen breakdown.

22. Signal transduction by receptors

Questions
- How are receptor subtypes defined pharmacologically?
- How may ligand–receptor interactions result in cellular responses?
- Why may the time for signal transduction be different for different receptors?

Classification of receptors

Receptors are classified according to the specific physiological signalling molecule (agonist) that they recognize (e.g. acetylcholine receptors). Further subclassification is made on the basis of their ability to be selectively activated by agonist molecules (e.g. nicotinic and muscarinic acetylcholine receptors). Subclassification is also often made on the basis of the affinity (a measure of tightness of binding) of a series of antagonists.

Signal transduction by receptors

Common mechanisms used to transduce an extracellular signal into an intracellular event include:

- membrane-bound receptors with integral ion channels: ligand-gated ion channels (Fig. 3.22.1A)
- membrane-bound receptors with integral enzyme activity (Fig. 3.22.1B and 3.22.2)
- membrane-bound receptors coupled to G-proteins (Fig. 3.22.1C)
- intracellular receptors.

Membrane-bound receptors with integral ion channels

Agonist binding to ligand-gated ion channels results in a change in conformation and opening of a gated channel within the receptor structure, which permits the flow of ions down an electrochemical gradient. This transduces the chemical signal into an electrical event at the plasma membrane.

Ligand-gated ion channels may also be present on intracellular membranes to respond to intracellular signals. For example, inositol 1,4,5-trisphosphate interaction with its receptors in the endoplasmic reticulum opens a Ca^{2+} channel that releases stored Ca^{2+} into the cytoplasm (Ch. 25).

Membrane-bound receptors with integral enzyme activity

Agonist binding to the extracellular domain of membrane-bound receptors with integral enzyme activity causes a conformational change that activates intrinsic enzyme activity within the cytoplasmic domain (Fig. 3.22.1B). Assembly of these transmembrane-spanning receptors as dimers is probably required for activity of all receptors in this group. Examples include the atrial natriuretic peptide (ANP) receptor, which is linked to guanylyl cyclase, and the growth factor receptors (e.g. insulin receptor), which are linked to tyrosine kinase.

ANP signals vasorelaxation through an enzyme-linked receptor. ANP is released from the atrium in response to atrial stretch (e.g. in response to volume expansion or cardiac failure) and acts on vascular smooth muscle to stimulate the production

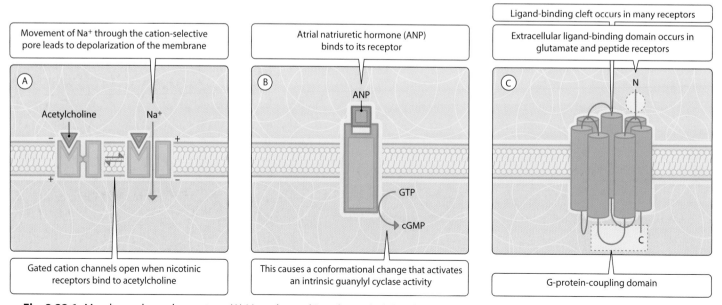

Fig. 3.22.1 Membrane-bound receptors. (A) Ligand-gated ion channels; (B) with intrinsic cytoplasmic enzyme activity; (C) coupled to G-proteins.

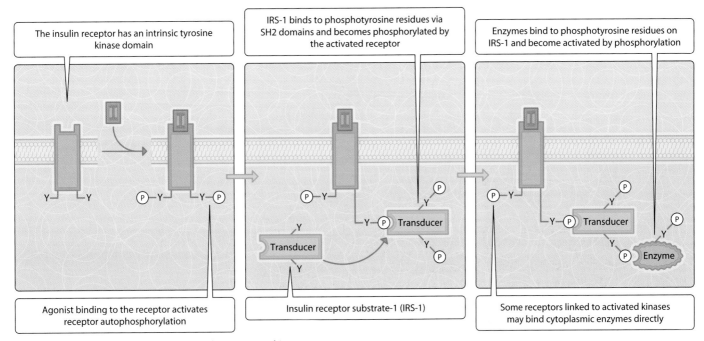

The insulin receptor has an intrinsic tyrosine kinase domain

IRS-1 binds to phosphotyrosine residues via SH2 domains and becomes phosphorylated by the activated receptor

Enzymes bind to phosphotyrosine residues on IRS-1 and become activated by phosphorylation

Agonist binding to the receptor activates receptor autophosphorylation

Insulin receptor substrate-1 (IRS-1)

Some receptors linked to activated kinases may bind cytoplasmic enzymes directly

Fig. 3.22.2 Membrane receptors linked to tyrosine kinase.

of the intracellular messenger cyclic GMP, leading to vaso-relaxation; the end result is a reduction in blood pressure.

Binding of hormone to extracellular binding sites in tyrosine kinase-linked receptors (Fig. 3.22.2) activates a kinase activity in the cytoplasmic domain of the receptor protein, which catalyses the transfer of a phosphate group from ATP onto tyrosine residues within its own structure (autophosphorylation). Phosphorylated residues are recognized either by transducing proteins (e.g. insulin receptor substrate-1) or directly by enzymes containing phosphotyrosine recognition sites: Src homology-2 (SH2) domains. On association with receptor or transducing protein, effector enzymes become activated allosterically or by phosphorylation by the receptor kinase, thus transducing the message into an intracellular chemical event.

Membrane-bound receptors coupled to G-proteins
The G-protein-coupled receptors have no integral enzyme or ion channel activity. They have seven transmembrane domains (7TMD) and couple to effector molecules via a transducing molecule, a GTP-binding regulatory protein (G-protein) (Fig. 3.22.1C). Effectors may be enzymes or ion channels. For example, in cardiac pacemaker cells, acetylcholine binding to M_2 muscarinic acetylcholine receptors inhibits adenylyl cyclase activity and stimulates K^+ channel opening via a G-protein, G_i. A wide variety of extracellular signalling molecules activate

G-protein-coupled receptors and, thus, there is an extensive superfamily of proteins with this common 7TMD structure. Often a number of different types of receptor exist for a particular agonist, each with its own pharmacology.

Intracellular receptors
Hydrophobic ligands, such as the steroid hormones cortisol, oestrogen and testosterone, penetrate the plasma membrane and bind to monomeric receptors in the cytoplasm or nucleus. In the resting state, these receptors are stabilized by association with heat shock or chaperone proteins. The activated receptor dissociates from the chaperone protein and translocates to the nucleus, where it binds to control regions in the DNA defined by specific sequences, thereby regulating gene expression. Cellular responses to intracellular receptor activation are relatively slow in onset because transcription and translation are required.

MYASTHENIA GRAVIS

Muscle weakness in patients with the autoimmune condition myasthenia gravis results from the presence of antibodies directed against nicotinic acetylcholine receptors. Binding of antibodies induces an increased rate of receptor degradation and the complement-dependent lysis of muscle fibres.

23. Transducing proteins

Questions
- How does the use of transducing proteins permit transient signalling?
- How do transducing proteins allow cells to integrate external signals?
- How is signal transduction modified by cholera toxin?

Many membrane receptors employ intermediary proteins to transduce the events of receptor activation to effector molecules in the cell (e.g. insulin receptor substrate-1 (Ch. 22) and GTP-binding regulatory proteins (G-proteins)).

Heteromeric GTP-binding regulatory proteins (G-proteins)

The heteromeric G-proteins are a large family of proteins that transduce the signal from receptors with seven transmembrane domains (7TMD; G-protein-coupled receptors) to a variety of effector molecules. Each G-protein has a common heterotrimeric structure of three distinct subunits: alpha (α), bound to GDP, beta (β) and gamma (γ). Receptor activation induces a conformational change in the G-protein. This change in structure causes the release of GDP and the binding of GTP in its place. The α-subunit carrying GTP (α-GTP) and the complex of βγ-subunits both dissociate from the receptor and go on to interact with, and activate or inhibit, specific effector molecules (Fig. 3.23.1). A slow integral GTPase activity in the α-subunit hydrolyses GTP and returns the α-subunit to its inactive conformation and α-GDPβγ heterotrimers reform. In this way, G-proteins act as a molecular switch (GDP/GTP exchange) to activate intracellular effector molecules but also as a timer (GTP hydrolysis) to ensure that the cellular activation is transient and occurs only while the extracellular signalling molecule is present at the cell surface.

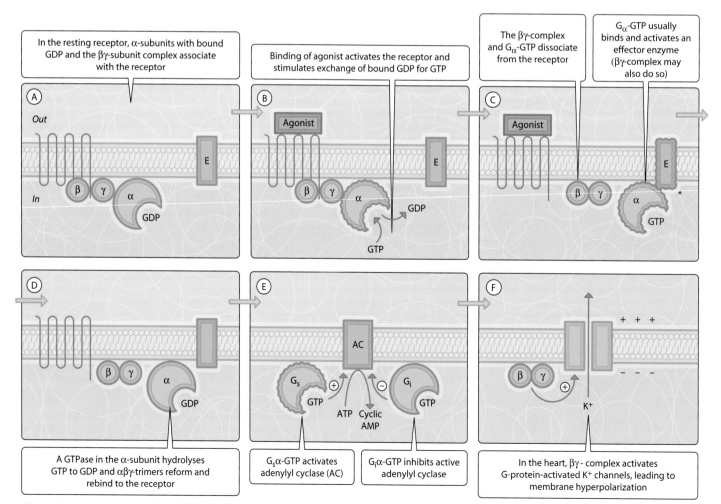

Fig. 3.23.1 G-protein-mediated signal transduction from receptor to effector.

G-protein diversity

G-protein coupling is a widely used mechanism with many permutations. Multiple isoforms of the α-, β- and γ-subunits have been identified. Different combinations of these can couple over 500 different receptors to at least 10 enzyme or ion channel effector molecules. The specificity of a G-protein is defined by the α-subunit present (Fig. 3.23.1). These include G_s (stimulates adenylyl cyclase), G_i (inhibits adenylyl cyclase), G_q (stimulates phospholipase C; Fig. 3.23.2) and G_t (transducin in retinal rod cells, which transduces the detection of light into enzyme activation).

Monomeric G-proteins

A second family of monomeric GTP-binding regulatory proteins was identified initially as products of viral oncogenes (cancer-inducing genes). A member of this family, **Ras**, is responsible for producing tumours of connective tissue (sarcomas). In normal cells, these G-proteins participate in signalling pathways involved in the transmission of signals from tyrosine kinase-linked receptors in pathways concerned with the regulation of cell growth and differentiation. However, unlike the trimeric G-proteins, the Ras proteins do not interact directly with the membrane receptor (Fig. 3.23.3).

Like the heterotrimeric G-protein α subunits, Ras proteins bind GDP in the inactive state and GTP when activated. In this case, nucleotide exchange is stimulated by guanine-nucleotide-releasing proteins (GNRPs), such as Grb2 and Sos. As with the trimeric G-proteins, Ras is inactivated on slow hydrolysis of GTP. This can be increased over 100-fold by the interaction of GTPase-activating proteins (GAP).

Ras couples tyrosine kinase receptor signalling to cell growth and differentiation. Other members of the Ras family couple tyrosine kinase receptor signalling to the cytoskeleton (Rho), vesicle transport (Rab (Ch. 15), ARF) and nuclear protein import (Ran1; Ch. 14).

SH2 and SH3 domains in adapter proteins

The Src homology domains SH2 and SH3 were initially identified in the product of the *src* oncogene. They are common in signalling pathway proteins and permit protein–protein association. The SH2 domains recognize phosphotyrosine residues within specific short sequences of amino acid residues and SH3 domains recognize amino acid sequences rich in proline residues.

CHOLERA AND WHOOPING COUGH

Cholera toxin covalently modifies $G_s\alpha$ with an ADP-ribosyl group from NAD^+. This modification inhibits the GTPase activity of $G_s\alpha$, resulting in constitutive activation of the G-protein. Pertussis toxin from the bacterium that produces whooping cough, *Bordetella pertussis*, covalently modifies $G_i\alpha$ with an ADP-ribosyl group that prevents receptor association. This modification inhibits the G_i inhibitory pathway, thereby leading to cellular activation through the unchecked action of G_s-activated pathways.

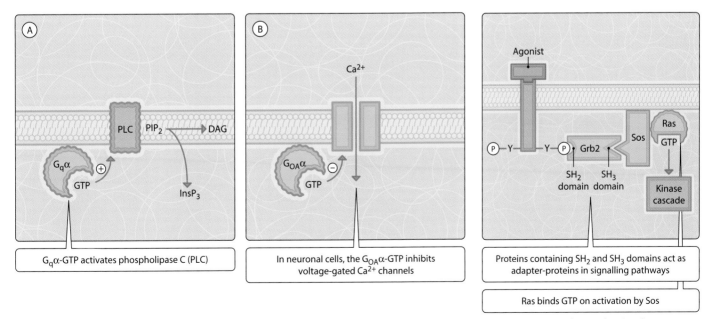

Fig. 3.23.2 The specificity of a G-protein is determined by its subunits. PIP_2, phosphatidylinositol 4,5-bisphosphate; $InsP_3$, inositol 1,4,5-trisphosphate; DAG, diacylglycerol.

Fig. 3.23.3 Signal transduction by adapter proteins.

$G_q\alpha$-GTP activates phospholipase C (PLC)

In neuronal cells, the $G_{OA}\alpha$-GTP inhibits voltage-gated Ca^{2+} channels

Proteins containing SH_2 and SH_3 domains act as adapter-proteins in signalling pathways

Ras binds GTP on activation by Sos

24. Second messengers

Questions
- What is a second messenger?
- What are the necessary properties of a second messenger?
- How do second messengers activate intracellular signalling pathways?

Activation of many receptors results in cascades of intracellular cell signalling events initiated through transducing proteins, intracellular (second) messengers and effector enzymes.

Characteristics of second messengers
In many instances, the response to receptor activation is activation of an enzyme effector, which produces a small intracellular messenger molecule or 'second messenger'. So that intracellular signalling occurs only during receptor activation, second messengers must:
- be maintained at low concentration in the resting cell
- be produced only in response to activation of specific receptors
- be produced in proportion to the size of the extracellular signal
- produce a cellular response in proportion to the change in concentration of the second messenger

- be degraded rapidly to ensure transience in signalling pathways.

Cyclic nucleotides
Cyclic adenosine 3',5'-monophosphate (cyclic AMP; Fig. 3.24.1) is produced by an integral plasma membrane enzyme, **adenylyl cyclase**, which converts ATP to cyclic AMP and pyrophosphate. Adenylyl cyclase is activated by receptors that couple through the G-protein G_s, while receptors coupling through G_i produce an inhibitory response. Cyclic AMP transmits the signal through the cytoplasm by diffusion to cyclic AMP-dependent protein kinase (cA-PK), which is then activated to phosphorylate a variety of target proteins within the cell, activating or inhibiting their activity. Cyclic AMP is rapidly hydrolysed by cellular **cyclic AMP phosphodiesterases**, which ensure a rapid return to basal levels once the extracellular stimulus is removed. Caffeine and theophylline both inhibit cyclic AMP phosphodiesterase and, therefore, act in synergy with adenylyl cyclase activation to produce a larger cyclic AMP response for a given extracellular signal.

Phospholipid-derived second messengers
A widely used substrate for the generation of second messengers is the minor phospholipid phosphatidylinositol 4,5-bisphosphate

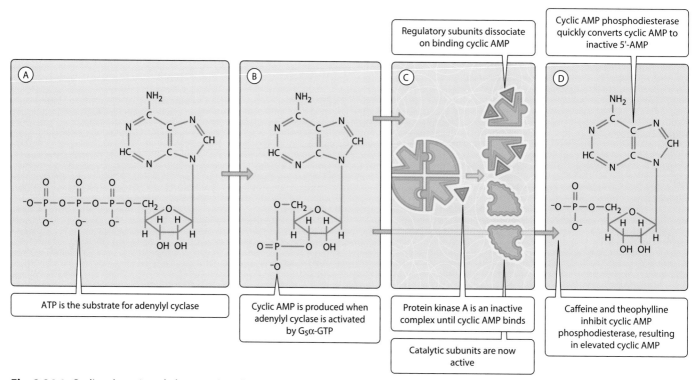

Fig. 3.24.1 Cyclic adenosine 3',5'-monophosphate (cyclic AMP) second messenger.

(PIP$_2$). Activation of PIP$_2$ phosphodiesterase (phospholipase C (PLC)) releases the phospholipid head group inositol 1,4,5-trisphosphate (InsP$_3$) leaving diacylglycerol (DAG) in the membrane (Fig. 3.24.2). The released InsP$_3$ diffuses in the cytoplasm to the endo(sarco)plasmic reticulum where it activates specific InsP$_3$-gated Ca^{2+} channels (InsP$_3$ receptors) to release stored Ca^{2+}. DAG acts within the membrane as an activator of protein kinase C by reducing its concentration dependence on [Ca^{2+}]$_i$. Thus, both hydrolysis products of PIP$_2$ are second messengers that activate downstream signalling elements.

In some cells, InsP$_3$ may be acted on by InsP$_3$ kinase to produce inositol 1,3,4,5-tetrakisphosphate (InsP$_4$), which represents a further putative second messenger (Fig. 3.24.3). InsP$_4$ may be involved in raising intracellular Ca^{2+} concentrations, either by facilitating the movement of Ca^{2+} between intracellular vesicular stores or by stimulating store refilling from the extracellular medium. The removal of InsP$_4$ is by degradation to inositol 1,3,4-trisphosphate (differing position of the phosphate groups to InsP$_3$), which does not stimulate the InsP$_3$ receptor or InsP$_4$-sensitive mechanisms.

In some cells, DAG production from alternative non-inositol phospholipids may also occur, giving a greater and prolonged response to certain agonists than can be provided by PIP$_2$ breakdown alone.

The InsP$_3$ signal is terminated by InsP$_3$ 5-phosphatase, to produce inositol 1,4-bisphosphate (InsP$_2$), which is inactive at InsP$_3$ receptors. Removal of DAG is either by conversion to monoacylglycerol or by the action of DAG kinase to form phosphatidic acid.

Local chemical mediators arising from phospholipid metabolism

Further oxidative metabolism of arachidonic acid, released in response to cell stimulation, via the eicosanoid pathways can result in the production of eicosanoids (leukotrienes, prostaglandins and thromboxanes). These molecules act as local chemical messengers, binding to specific receptors in adjacent cells to give a concerted tissue response.

THE NON-STEROIDAL ANTI-INFLAMMATORY DRUGS

The anti-inflammatory action of non-steroidal anti-inflammatory drugs (NSAIDs), such as aspirin (acetyl salicylate), paracetamol, ibuprofen and indometacin, is mediated predominantly by inhibition of prostaglandin G/H synthetase (cyclooxygenase), which reduces autocoid signalling via the synthesis and release of prostaglandins. For example, by decreasing circulating prostaglandins (e.g. PGE$_2$, PGI$_2$), NSAIDs reduce blood flow to inflamed tissue and, thereby, contribute to reduced oedema. This mechanism is also probably associated with the effectiveness of NSAIDs in relieving headache.

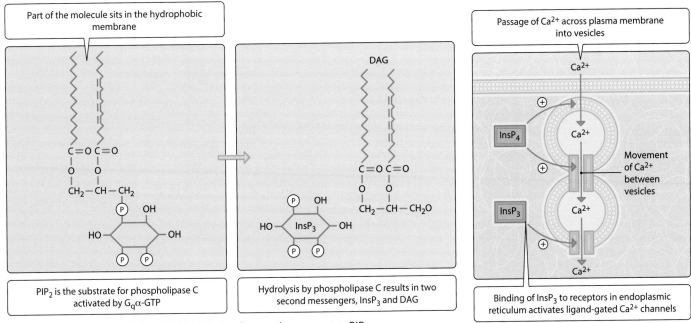

Fig. 3.24.2 Formation of phospholipid-derived second messengers. PIP$_2$, phosphatidylinositol 4,5-bisphosphate; InsP$_3$, inositol 1,4,5-trisphosphate; DAG, diacylglycerol.

Fig. 3.24.3 Action of inositol 1,4,5-trisphosphate (InsP$_3$).

25. Calcium ions as a second messenger

Questions
- How is intracellular free Ca^{2+} concentration, $[Ca^{2+}]_i$, maintained at submicromolar concentrations?
- How do cells achieve a controlled increase in $[Ca^{2+}]_i$?
- How do Ca^{2+}-responsive mechanisms maintain specificity to micromolar Ca^{2+} when cellular Mg^{2+} is millimolar?

Cellular Ca^{2+} metabolism

A variety of cellular responses are mediated by changes in the concentration of cytosolic Ca^{2+} (e.g. contraction, secretion, glycogenolysis). Binding of Ca^{2+} induces conformational changes in Ca^{2+}-sensitive proteins that modulate their activity. Cells go to great lengths to maintain extremely low (100–200 nmol/l) cytosolic Ca^{2+} concentrations ($[Ca^{2+}]_i$) in spite of the large electrochemical gradient (10 000:1), which favours strongly the influx of Ca^{2+} from the interstitial fluid (1–2 mmol/l) (Fig. 3.25.1). Although there is limited buffering of Ca^{2+} by binding to intracellular proteins, cells need to expend energy to extrude Ca^{2+} through the plasma membrane or to sequester it in intracellular vesicular stores. Indeed, total cell $[Ca^{2+}]$ can be in the millimolar range when stored Ca^{2+} is taken into account. Extrusion occurs via Ca^{2+}-ATPase and Na^+–Ca^{2+} exchangers in the plasma membrane and sequestration into intracellular vesicular stores via the sarco(endo)plasmic reticulum Ca^{2+}-ATPase (SERCA) (Fig. 3.25.1). In the lumen of these stores, the free $[Ca^{2+}]$ is buffered by binding to low-affinity Ca^{2+}-binding proteins (e.g. calsequestrin). This reduces the unfavourable gradient for further Ca^{2+} uptake and allows a considerable total concentration (in the millimolar range) to be stored. Uptake into mitochondria, driven by the large membrane potential from proton extrusion, can also occur to buffer Ca^{2+} during prolonged periods of significantly raised $[Ca^{2+}]_i$.

Transient, 5–10-fold, increases in total $[Ca^{2+}]_i$ occur in response to cell activation and may be mediated by influx across the plasma membrane or release from intracellular stores (Fig. 3.25.2). In both cases, the movement of Ca^{2+} across the membrane is driven by the electrochemical gradient through one or more Ca^{2+}-specific ion channels. These may be directly ligand-gated (e.g. N-methyl-D-aspartate (NMDA) receptors in the plasma membrane and inositol 1,4,5-trisphosphate (InsP$_3$) receptors in the ER) or may open in response to changes in membrane potential (e.g. voltage-gated Ca^{2+} channels in the plasma membrane; Ch. 19). In addition, Ca^{2+} itself may stimulate opening of InsP$_3$-receptor channels and a second related channel, the 'ryanodine receptor'.

Owing to the limited diffusion of Ca^{2+} in the cytoplasm, Ca^{2+} transients are often localized to microdomains within the cell (e.g. below the plasma membrane), where the $[Ca^{2+}]_i$ may rise to 100–200 µmol/l (e.g. to trigger exocytosis).

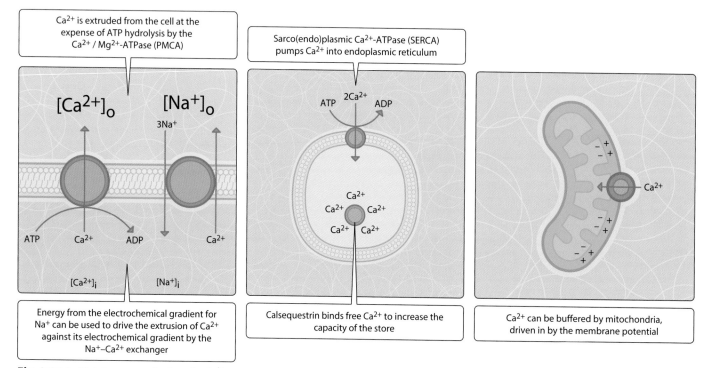

Fig. 3.25.1 Maintenance of cytosolic Ca^{2+} concentrations.

Capacitance entry of Ca²⁺

Mobilized Ca^{2+} from internal stores may be resequestered by the ER or may be pumped out of the cell by plasma membrane Ca^{2+}-ATPases. In principle, this latter mechanism could lead to depletion of the Ca^{2+} store. In practice, reduced lumenal $[Ca^{2+}]$ in the ER (SR) stimulates a refilling of internal Ca^{2+} stores from extracellular sources by store-operated Ca^{2+} channels (Fig. 3.25.2C). Such refilling of internal Ca^{2+} stores is known as capacitance entry of Ca^{2+}.

Proteins modulated by Ca²⁺

Some Ca^{2+}-sensitive proteins contain the Ca^{2+}-binding site in the same polypeptide as the protein activity (e.g. protein kinase C). Many Ca^{2+}-sensitive proteins, however, employ independent Ca^{2+}-binding protein subunits to confer Ca^{2+} sensitivity. **Calmodulin** is most often employed; this is a small polypeptide containing four Ca^{2+}-binding sites in each molecule that are highly selective for Ca^{2+} over Na^+, K^+ and Mg^{2+}. Large conformational changes in the calmodulin molecule are induced by the successive binding of pairs of Ca^{2+}. In most cases, interaction of calmodulin with target proteins occurs only after activation of calmodulin by binding Ca^{2+}, although in some cases calmodulin remains tightly bound to the target enzyme even at resting Ca^{2+} concentrations (e.g. glycogen phosphorylase).

THE USE OF CALCIUM ANTAGONISTS IN CARDIOVASCULAR DISEASE

The calcium antagonists (Ca^{2+} entry blockers) are drugs that act selectively on the cardiovascular system to block L-type, voltage-gated Ca^{2+} channels and so reduce Ca^{2+} entry and, thereby, contractile activity. Vascular selective dihydropyridines are indicated in hypertension to lower vascular smooth muscle tone and, hence, blood pressure. In angina, the ischaemic heart can be treated with dihydropyridines and diltiazem to improve the coronary circulation, by reducing coronary artery contraction, and to reduce cardiac oxygen consumption, by reducing contractile activity.

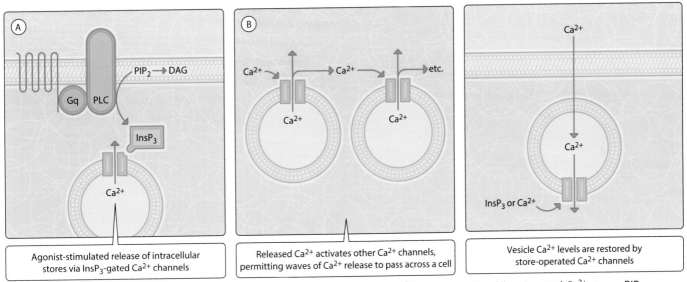

Fig. 3.25.2 Achieving transient changes in intracellular Ca^{2+}. (A,B) Increasing Ca^{2+} in cytosol; (C) refilling internal Ca^{2+} stores. PIP_2, phosphatidylinositol 4,5-bisphosphate; $Ins\,P_3$, inositol 1,4,5-trisphosphate; DAG, diacylglycerol; PLC, phospholipase C.

26. Kinases and phosphatases in cell signalling

Questions
- How is protein activity regulated by phosphorylation and dephosphorylation?
- How are the activities of protein kinases and phosphatases controlled?
- If many second messengers control the activity of a protein kinase, how is the specificity of different cellular signals maintained?

Regulation of enzyme and protein activity is often achieved by phosphorylation or dephosphorylation directed. The presence of a negatively charged phosphate group at specific residues in the target protein affects the conformation of the polypeptide, which can cause either activation or inhibition depending on the protein.

Phosphorylation

Protein kinases
Protein kinases transfer the terminal phosphate from ATP onto residues containing a hydroxyl group within a specific consensus amino acid sequence. Most protein phosphorylation is catalysed by serine and theonine kinases with only a small proportion (0.1%) catalysed by tyrosine kinases.

All protein kinases have regulatory and catalytic elements. These may be contained on separate polypeptide subunits (e.g. cyclic AMP-dependent protein kinase (cA-PK)) (Fig. 3.26.1) or combined in a single polypeptide (e.g. protein kinase C). Protein kinase C is maintained in an inactive form by binding of a regulatory domain with a pseudosubstrate motif to block the active site of the catalytic domain. Binding of diacylglycerol (DAG) and Ca^{2+} induces a conformational change that unmasks the active site. In the absence of regulator molecules, protein kinases are inactive. Activation occurs on interaction with the regulatory element of the regulator molecule (second messenger) or by phosphorylation/dephosphorylation, which induces a conformational change to render the catalytic site accessible to substrate.

Where a subset of cellular proteins is modulated by a single kinase, their activities are often modulated in concert. For example, in hepatic glycogen metabolism, breakdown is increased while synthesis is reduced in response to cA-PK activation, producing a concerted mobilization of glucose (Fig. 3.26.2).

Many target proteins contain more than one phosphorylation site, presenting the potential for signal integration. These may represent (a) multiple sites for a single protein kinase, (b) single sites phosphorylated by more than one kinase or (c) specific

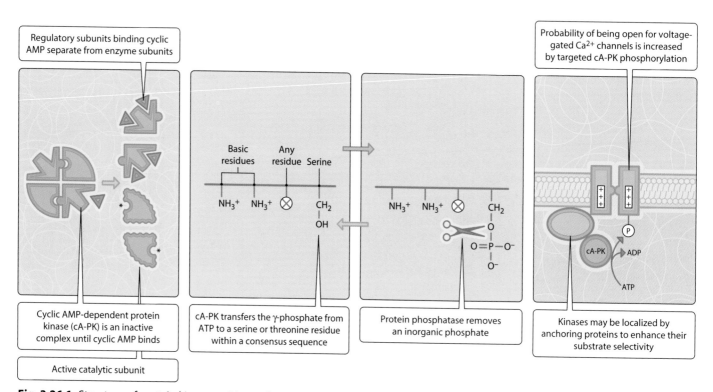

Fig. 3.26.1 Structure of protein kinases, with regulatory and catalytic elements. cA-PK, cyclic AMP-dependent protein kinase.

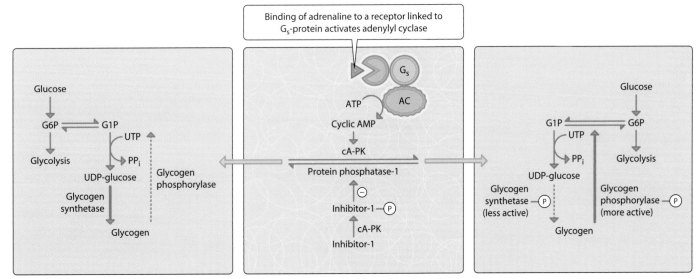

Fig. 3.26.2 Concerted action of cyclic AMP-dependent protein kinase (cA-PK) in mobilization of glycogen stores.

sites for different kinases. Phosphorylation at multiple sites may alter the activity of the protein but could also modulate the phosphorylation or response to phosphorylation at one of the other sites.

Autophosphorylation

Most protein kinases are able to catalyse self-phosphorylation or autophosphorylation, which is important for self-regulation. For example, autophosphorylation of Ca^{2+}-calmodulin-dependent protein kinase abolishes the calmodulin dependence of the enzyme. Autophosphorylation of the insulin receptor kinase results in an activation of the kinase, which is then independent of the binding of insulin. In the receptors linked to tyrosine kinases, autophosphorylation is additionally important as the resulting phosphotyrosine residues provide interaction sites for effector molecules and transducing proteins (Ch. 22).

Dephosphorylation: phosphoprotein phosphatases

Protein phosphatases catalyse the hydrolysis of phosphate bonds (dephosphorylation) and may be classified into serine (threonine) and tyrosine phosphatases. Many protein phosphatases are cytoplasmic; however, one class of membrane-bound tyrosine phosphatase probably acts as receptors and has been implicated in intracellular signalling in leukocytes in response to adhesion proteins and antigen.

Cross-talk between signalling pathways

Signalling pathways do not operate independently; rather there is considerable cross-talk between them, which allows pathways to modulate each other. This permits a cell to integrate its response to multiple extracellular signals and, thus, to produce an appropriate overall response. The exact nature of the response in any cell will depend partly on the size of each external signal but also on the nature of the signalling pathway components present in the cell.

Targeting proteins for components of signalling pathways: molecular scaffolds

Kinases and phosphatases may be compartmentalized within the cell by association with subcellular targeting proteins associated with membrane structures. Targeting can increase the selectivity of broad-specificity kinases or phosphatases by favouring their access to particular substrates. Several anchoring proteins have been characterized that localize kinases and phosphatases to different cellular localizations. Further complexity is possible when the targeting protein is able to bind several kinases and/or phosphatases, providing a molecular scaffold to localize signalling enzymes. An example of a scaffold protein is A-kinase-anchoring protein 79 (AKAP79), which targets cA-PK, protein kinase C and protein phosphatase-2B to the post-synaptic density of mammalian synapses. In this way, molecular scaffolds can provide for the integrated response of an effector to several second messenger pathways.

27. Desensitization (tachyphylaxis) in signalling pathways

Questions
- What is desensitization?
- What is the difference between homologous and heterologous desensitization?
- By what mechanisms may adrenoceptors become desensitized?
- How may cells develop supersensitivity to extracellular signalling molecules?

When cells are exposed continuously to an extracellular messenger or drug, they can often become increasingly resistant to stimu-lation. This loss of sensitivity is known as desensitization or tachyphylaxis when it occurs acutely over a few minutes, and tolerance or resistance when occurring over a period of days or weeks. Desensitization can take two forms. When sensitivity is lost to a single extracellular agonist, this is known as homologous desensitization (Fig. 3.27.1). When sensitivity is lost to multiple stimulating agonists in response to the presence of a single stimulating agonist, this is known as heterologous desensitization (Fig. 3.27.2).

Many mechanisms may contribute to cellular desensitization. At the level of the receptor, a change in receptor properties or a

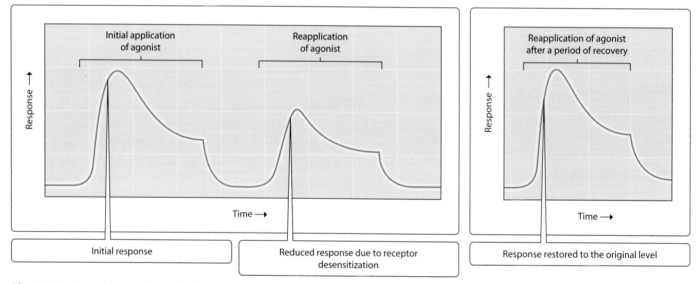

Fig. 3.27.1 Homologous desensitization.

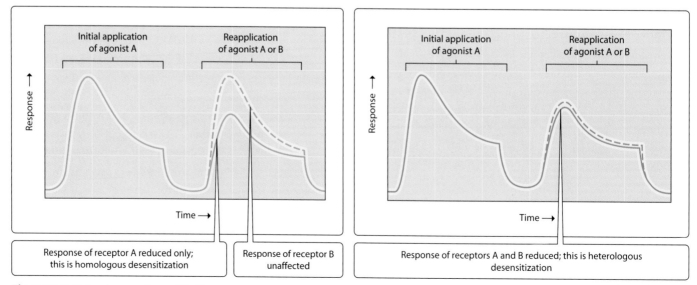

Fig. 3.27.2 Heterologous desensitization.

reduction in the number of receptors may bring about desensitization. Alternatively, metabolic desensitization could occur through exhaustion of a mediator within a signalling pathway, increased degradation of the extracellular signalling molecule and/or physiological adaptation to the raised levels of signalling molecule.

Receptor desensitization

Ligand-gated ion channels desensitize rapidly. When continually exposed to agonist, these receptors undergo a slow transition to a stable conformation that binds agonist with high affinity but in which the channel remains closed. Desensitization is reversed when the concentration of agonist falls and the agonist dissociates.

Desensitization of G-protein-coupled receptors can occur through modification of the activated receptor by phosphorylation, reversible removal of the receptor from the plasma membrane or irreversible removal and degradation of the receptor; the last is known as **downregulation**. Receptor phosphorylation may be in response to protein kinases activated by second messengers (e.g. cyclic AMP-dependent protein kinase (cA-PK) or protein kinase C) or specific G-protein-receptor protein kinases (e.g. β-adrenoceptor kinase) (Fig. 3.27.3).

Some activated receptors can be internalized by receptor-mediated endocytosis. A short period of desensitization results if the internalized receptors are sorted and recycled to the plasma membrane. On prolonged cell stimulation, receptors may become targeted to lysosomes where they are degraded; this results in receptor downregulation. The results of downregulation are reversed only by the synthesis of new receptors. It is noteworthy that downregulation of receptors can occur in response to molecules other than agonist. For example, ethanol and barbiturates, which are not receptor agonists, may lead to downregulation of G-protein-coupled receptors, an example of **tolerance**.

Cell supersensitivity

The sensitivity of a cell to an external stimulus may be increased by convergent cross-talk between signalling pathways. For example, glucagon and glucagon-like peptide do not stimulate release of insulin from beta-cells per se but potentiate the response to a given level of glucose through a cA-PK mechanism. Similarly, β-adrenergic stimulation in the heart can increase heart rate and force of contraction, again through a cA-PK mechanism via phosphorylation of L-type voltage-sensitive Ca^{2+} channels. This phosphorylation increases the probability that Ca^{2+} channels will open and, therefore, leads to a greater Ca^{2+} signal for a given depolarization.

Supersensitivity may also occur following interruption of normal signalling to the cell. This is often seen after denervation of peripheral tissues. The response in the postsynaptic cell can be to increase the number of receptors and to increase post-junctional responsiveness by increasing electrical excitability.

RECEPTOR DESENSITIZATION AND INSULIN RESISTANCE IN DIABETES

In type 2 diabetes mellitus, tissues become resistant to insulin even though insulin may be present at raised levels. One contributory factor to insulin resistance is the downregulation of insulin receptors.

DRUG HABITUATION AND 'REBOUND' EFFECTS

Habituation to drugs
Downregulation in general may explain habituation to drug therapy.

Rebound effects on removal of drug therapy
Adaptive responses in cells in an attempt to overcome the effect of a drug during treatment may result in a rebound effect in response to natural agonists when therapy ceases. For example, sudden withdrawal of β-adrenoceptor antagonists can cause an increased sympathetic stimulation of the heart. The resulting increase in heart rate and force of contraction, and hence oxygen consumption, can lead to the development of angina pectoris and myocardial infarction.

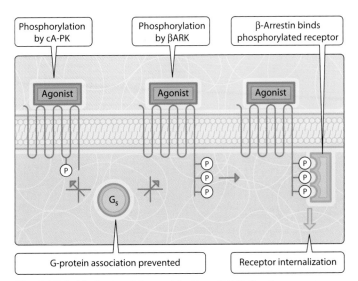

Fig. 3.27.3 Methods of desensitization. βARK, β-adrenoceptor kinase; cA-PK, cyclic AMP-dependent protein kinase.

28. Neurotransmission

Questions
- How are messages passed between nerve cells?
- How is electrical activity coupled to neurotransmitter release?
- How is neurotransmitter recognition translated into a postsynaptic response?
- What is the difference between fast and slow neurotransmission?

Fast electrical transmission
The passage of an electrical signal between cells can only occur when two cells are tightly physically coupled by gap junctions (e.g. in cardiac and smooth muscles).

Chemical (synaptic) transmission
Chemical transmission of information between excitable cells occurs at specialized junctions called synapses. A chemical transmitter is released from the presynaptic structure of the signalling cell in response to depolarization and the influx of Ca^{2+} (Fig. 3.28.1). The transmitter molecule diffuses across the synaptic cleft and binds to a specific receptor molecule on the postsynaptic cell, where it elicits a response (Fig. 3.28.2).

Neurotransmitter release
In nerve cells, neurotransmitters are stored in, and released from, vesicular stores in the presynaptic nerve terminal. Release is, therefore, quantal in nature, each quantum representing the contents of one vesicle. On excitation, the rise in $[Ca^{2+}]_i$ triggers release of vesicle attachments to the cytoskeleton and synaptic vesicle docking and fusion at the presynaptic membrane. There is a small delay (0.5 ms) between the arrival of the action potential and the response in the postsynaptic cell owing to the time taken for transmitter release, diffusion across the synapse and postsynaptic receptor activation.

Postsynaptic potentials
Chemical transmission can be fast or slow. The response in the cell may be excitatory or inhibitory.

Fast synaptic neurotransmission
In fast synaptic transmission (millisecond time range), agonist binding results directly in the opening of an integral ion channel in the receptor (ionotropic receptor) and, thereby, a change in membrane potential.

Excitatory neurotransmission
Excitatory transmitters open channels for ions with positive equilibrium potentials (Na^+, Ca^{2+}) resulting in membrane depolarization (excitatory postsynaptic potentials) (Ch. 17). Such potentials may bring the adjacent membrane containing voltage-gated channels to the threshold for action potential generation in the postsynaptic cell (e.g. nicotinic acetylcholine receptor activation).

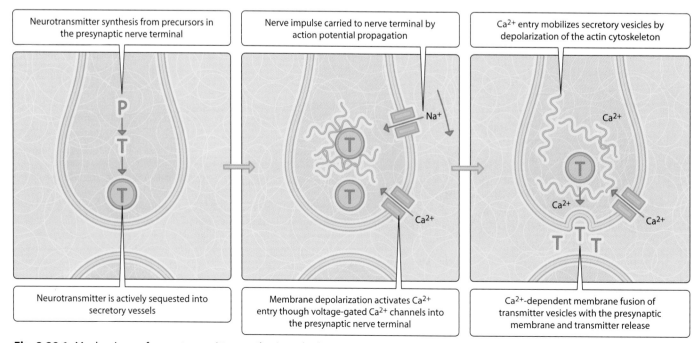

Neurotransmitter synthesis from precursors in the presynaptic nerve terminal

Nerve impulse carried to nerve terminal by action potential propagation

Ca^{2+} entry mobilizes secretory vesicles by depolarization of the actin cytoskeleton

Neurotransmitter is actively sequested into secretory vessels

Membrane depolarization activates Ca^{2+} entry though voltage-gated Ca^{2+} channels into the presynaptic nerve terminal

Ca^{2+}-dependent membrane fusion of transmitter vesicles with the presynaptic membrane and transmitter release

Fig. 3.28.1 Mechanisms of neurotransmitter synthesis and release.

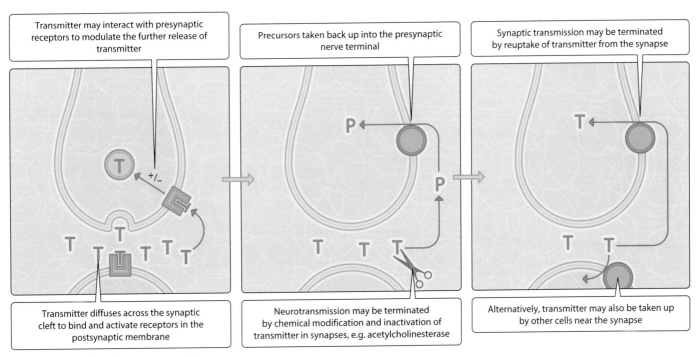

Transmitter may interact with presynaptic receptors to modulate the further release of transmitter

Precursors taken back up into the presynaptic nerve terminal

Synaptic transmission may be terminated by reuptake of transmitter from the synapse

Transmitter diffuses across the synaptic cleft to bind and activate receptors in the postsynaptic membrane

Neurotransmission may be terminated by chemical modification and inactivation of transmitter in synapses, e.g. acetylcholinesterase

Alternatively, transmitter may also be taken up by other cells near the synapse

Fig. 3.28.2 Action of neurotransmitters.

At the neuromuscular junction, small spontaneous postsynaptic potential changes of 0.5–1.0 mV can be observed under resting conditions. These miniature endplate potentials result from the release from the presynaptic nerve terminal of a single vesicle (quantum) of acetylcholine and are too small to trigger an action potential in the muscle.

Inhibitory neurotransmission

Inhibitory transmitters (e.g. glycine or gama-aminobutyric acid (GABA)) open channels for ions with negative equilibrium potentials (K^+, Cl^-) resulting in membrane hyperpolarization (inhibitory postsynaptic potential) and, thereby, reduced membrane excitability.

Slow synaptic neurotransmission

In slow synaptic transmission (seconds to hours), the receptor (metabotropic receptor) signals to channel proteins via G-proteins within the membrane either directly or indirectly via intracellular second messenger molecules or kinases.

Termination of neurotransmission

Neurotransmission is terminated by removal of the transmitter from the synapse, either by degradation (e.g. acetylcholinesterase) or by reuptake into the presynaptic nerve terminal or an adjacent cell via specific transporters (e.g. for noradrenaline).

MICROBIAL TOXINS ACTING ON NEUROTRANSMISSION

Botulinum and tetanus toxins produce quite different clinical symptoms of parasympathetic and motor paralysis, and prolonged convulsions, respectively. Both toxins act presynaptically to cleave specific components of the SNARE ternary complexes, which target secretory vesicles to the synapse, thereby reducing transmitter release. Botulinum toxin inhibits acetylcholine release specifically, while tetanus toxin reduces inhibitory amino acid transmitter release in the spinal cord. It is noteworthy that local injection of botulinum toxin can be used clinically to treat local muscle spasm.

NEUROMUSCULAR BLOCKING DRUGS IN ANAESTHESIA

Reflex movements in patients during surgery are commonly inhibited using two classes of drug that block the action of acetylcholine.

- Competitive antagonists bind to nicotinic acetylcholine receptors in competition with acetylcholine and prevent channel opening (e.g. (+)-tubocurarine, gallamine and pancuronium).
- Depolarizing blockers (e.g. succinylcholine) act as nicotinic agonists, initially opening the channel. The resulting membrane depolarization causes Na^+ channels to open and inactivate, producing a rapid 'phase I' block of neurotransmission. Over a period of time (minutes), the electrical excitability of the muscle membrane is restored as it repolarizes. However, neurotransmission remains blocked (phase II) as the continued presence of the blocker produces receptor desensitization (Ch. 27).

29. Glucose-stimulated insulin release from beta-cells

Questions

- How is glucose concentration coupled to electrical excitation in beta-cells of the islets of Langerhans?
- How is electrical excitation in the beta-cell coupled to the release of insulin?
- How may drugs stimulate insulin release from beta-cells?

Mechanism

Glucose-stimulated insulin release from beta-cells of the pancreatic islets of Langerhans depends on the coupling of metabolism to the modification of ion channel activity. Glucose uptake and entry into glycolysis is proportional to the circulating glucose concentration because of the high K_M values of the GLUT2 glucose transporter and the first enzyme in the glycolytic pathway, glucokinase (Fig. 3.29.1). The internalized glucose is

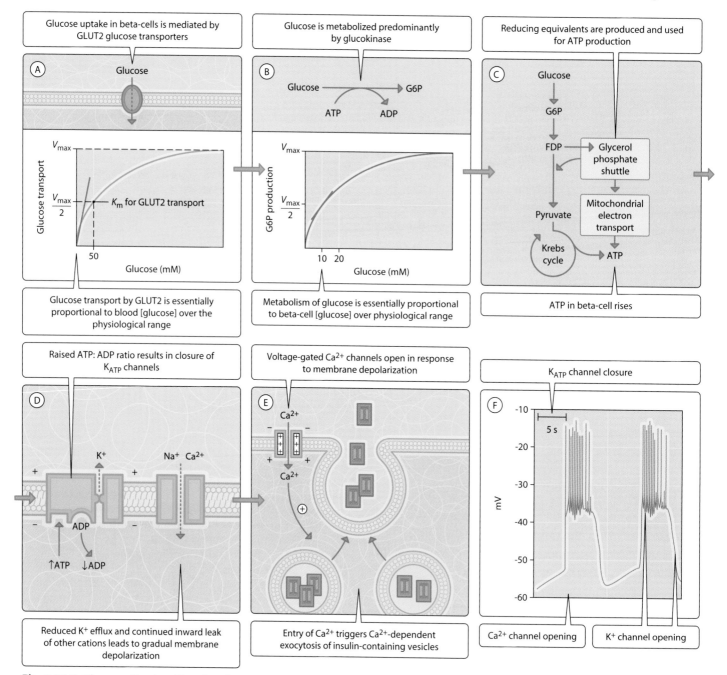

Fig. 3.29.1 Glucose-stimulated insulin release. DHAP, dihydroxyacetone phosphate; FDP, fructose 1,6-bisphosphate; FAD, flavin adenine dinucleotide; NAD, nicotinamide adenine dinucleotide.

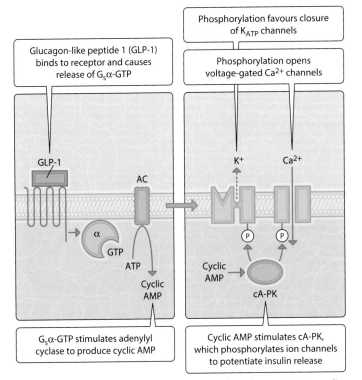

Fig. 3.29.2 Hormone potentiation of insulin release. cA-PK, cyclic AMP-dependent protein kinase.

then metabolized rapidly with the concomitant production of ATP. In the resting beta-cell, active ATP-sensitive K^+ (K_{ATP}) channels contribute to the resting membrane potential (Ch. 17). These channels close in response to raised ATP concentration and falling ADP concentration (Fig. 3.29.1D). This results in a gradual membrane depolarization and activation of L-type voltage-gated Ca^{2+} channels. A burst of action potentials follows, the length of which is proportional to the glucose concentration. Entry of Ca^{2+} during these bursts raises $[Ca^{2+}]_i$ and triggers the exocytosis of insulin-containing secretory vesicles (Fig. 3.29.1E). In addition to the repolarizing influence of activated delayed rectifier K^+ channels during each action potential, the raised $[Ca^{2+}]_i$ also stimulates the opening of Ca^{2+}-sensitive K^+ channels, which contribute to the repolarization of the membrane at the end of the bursts (Fig. 3.29.1F).

Insulin is synthesized as a proinsulin precursor and is only processed to mature insulin in the secretory vesicle. This prevents inappropriate activation of insulin receptors that may be present in the endoplasmic reticulum.

Potentiators and inhibitors of insulin secretion

Although not direct stimulators of insulin secretion, hormones such as glucagon (signalling metabolic stress) and glucagon-like peptide 1 (GLP-1; signalling arrival of a food bolus in the gut) potentiate glucose-stimulated insulin secretion (Fig. 3.29.2). Signalling by these hormones is via cyclic AMP and the activation

of cyclic AMP-dependent protein kinase (cA-PK). Resulting phosphorylation of ion channels and other mechanisms involved in stimulus–secretion coupling increase the response to a given concentration of glucose, through closure of K_{ATP} channels, activation of voltage-gated Ca^{2+} channels and sensitization of the secretory machinery. These hormones do not stimulate insulin secretion on their own, as they require Ca^{2+}-calmodulin complex formation for the activation of cA-PK.

In contrast, some hormones, such as noradrenaline, somatostatin and prostaglandins, act to inhibit insulin secretion. Inhibition is mediated through signalling pathways activated by the G-proteins G_i and G_o acting to antagonize the excitation–secretion mechanism. Activation of signalling through the G_i family inhibits the downstream secretory machinery; G_o inhibits voltage-gated Ca^{2+} channels, and both G_i and G_o activate K_{ATP} channels.

Diabetes mellitus

Type 1 diabetes mellitus
Type 1 diabetes mellitus arises mostly in young people and is caused by the autoimmune destruction of insulin-producing beta-cells following infiltration of the islets of Langerhans by lymphoid cells. There is a strong genetic association with certain histocompatibility antigen (HLA) loci (DR3, DR4, DQ1, DQ8), indicating, perhaps, that in susceptible individuals inappropriate antigen presentation of normally sequestered self-antigens or of cross-reactive antigens following viral infection may lead to the onset of the disease. The HLA locus and other polymorphic gene loci that have been shown to have type 1 diabetes association suggest that immunological self-tolerance may have developed abnormally in these patients.

Type 2 diabetes mellitus
Type 2 diabetes mellitus develops in later adulthood. It is a progressive disease initiated by resistance to insulin in peripheral tissues, which becomes compounded by a failure in insulin secretion. During the development of the disease, raised circulating glucose concentrations put an increased demand on beta-cell insulin production. This may be aggravated by inhibition of glucose-sensing mechanisms through non-specific glycosylation and/or genetic susceptibility in the glucose-sensing mechanism

Ion channel modulation in the treatment of type 2 diabetes mellitus
Sulphonylurea K_{ATP} channel blockers (e.g. glibenclamide) trigger insulin release by producing a membrane depolarization in the absence of glucose. This class of drugs is used in patients with mild type 2 diabetes mellitus to overcome their hyperglycaemia and insulin resistance by raising endogenous insulin secretion.

30. Physical interactions between cells

Questions
- How do cells connect with each other and their environment physically?
- What type of molecules is involved in physical interactions?
- How do myocytes synchronize their contraction?

Adhesion molecules

The development and function of tissues is dependent on the physical interaction of one cell with another. These physical interactions are mediated by members of several families of membrane-spanning proteins, called adhesion molecules (Fig. 3.30.1). Adhesion molecules also play important roles in more transient interactions between cells, including those involved in cellular migration and the interactions between cells of the immune system.

Cadherins

Cells in a suspension made from different tissues tend to sort according to their origins: a property attributed to the patterns of expression of a family of universal calcium-dependent adhesion molecules called cadherins, which mediate homotypic cell–cell adhesion. Structurally, all cadherins have five extracellular domains and an intracellular domain that binds to complexes of cytoplasmic plaque proteins to form a link with the actin cytoskeleton or intermediate filaments. The linking of the cytoskeletons of neighbouring cells to form transcellular networks allows the formation of strong structures such as epithelial sheets.

Integrins

Cells not only interact physically with each other but also with the extracellular matrix (ECM). A second family of adhesion molecules, the **integrins**, are responsible for many of the interactions between cells and the ECM. Integrins are membrane-anchored heterodimeric glycoproteins. Each one consists of non-covalently associated α- and β-subunits. So far, 24 different combinations of α- and β-subunits have been identified in vivo. Both integrin subunits have cytoplasmic domains that are important for signal transduction and the formation of anchoring junctions. In addition to mediating cell–matrix interactions, a subgroup of integrins (those containing the β_2-subunit) can also form cell–cell interactions by acting as counter-receptors (ligands) for a third class of adhesion molecules, members of the immunoglobulin superfamily. The diversity of adhesive contacts formed by integrins means that they do not simply hold tissues together but also contribute to a wide range of physiological processes including cell migration, wound healing, inflammation, phagocytosis, platelet aggregation and T cell functions.

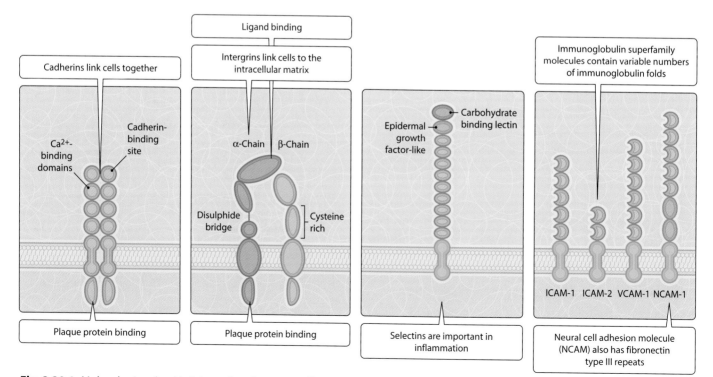

Fig. 3.30.1 Molecules involved in interactions between cells.

Immunoglobulin superfamily

The immunoglobulin superfamily is a large, diverse family of proteins that includes several adhesion molecules. In addition to acting as counter-receptors for β_2-integrins, molecules of the immunoglobulin superfamily on one cell may bind to identical molecules on another cell (homotypic binding), and to other members of the family (heterotypic binding). Family members, known as cellular adhesion molecules, play important roles in T cell interactions (intercellular adhesion molecule 1, ICAM-1) and in the binding of leukocytes to activated (ICAM-1; vascular adhesion molecule 1, VCAM-1) and resting (ICAM-2) endothelium. One of the most widely expressed immuno-globulin superfamily molecule is neural cell adhesion molecule (NCAM), which appears to play an important role in the developing nervous system.

Lectins

The lectins are a group of proteins recognizing carbohydrate ligands; the group includes the **selectins**, which are important in the recruitment of leukocytes to sites of inflammation, and a group of macrophage pattern recognition receptors, which bind to pathogens as part of inate immunity.

Gap junctions

Gap junctions are pores that link the cytoplasm of adjacent cells together. These pores are large enough to allow molecules up to 1000 Da to pass freely from cell to cell. This is sufficient to allow the passage of inorganic ions (Na^+, K^+, Ca^{2+}) and small organic molecules such as amino acids or second messengers (e.g. cyclic AMP, cyclic GMP or inositol 1,4,5-trisphosphate), but not macromolecules such as proteins or nucleic acids. These connections between cells mean that they can be coupled both chemically (or metabolically) and electrically. This helps a tissue to respond as an integrated unit rather than as individual cells. For example, it is important in synchronizing the contraction of myocytes to produce a beat in cardiac muscle. Like ion channels, gap junctions can be gated, i.e. their opening is regulated, by intracellular pH and Ca^{2+}.

 GENETIC DEFECTS AFFECTING ADHESION MOLECULES

Adhesion molecules play key roles in the migration of leukocytes to an inflammatory focus (Fig. 3.30.2). Genetic defects that lead to the loss of β_2-integrins or selectin ligands predispose affected individuals to recurrent infections.

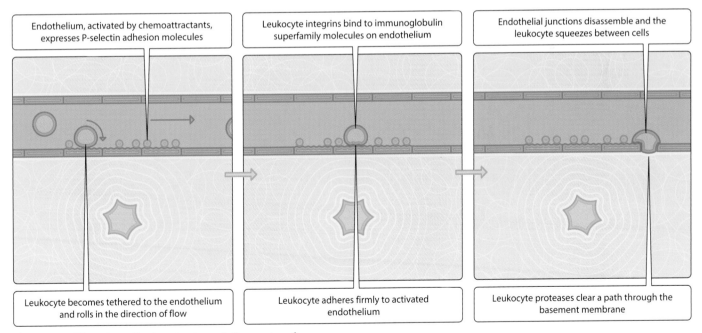

Endothelium, activated by chemoattractants, expresses P-selectin adhesion molecules

Leukocyte integrins bind to immunoglobulin superfamily molecules on endothelium

Endothelial junctions disassemble and the leukocyte squeezes between cells

Leukocyte becomes tethered to the endothelium and rolls in the direction of flow

Leukocyte adheres firmly to activated endothelium

Leukocyte proteases clear a path through the basement membrane

Fig. 3.30.2 Migration of leukocytes to an inflammatory focus.

31. Organization of cells into tissues

Questions
- How are the individual cells in a tissue organized?
- How can cells join together to form strong structures?
- How can cells anchor themselves to the extracellular matrix?

Tissues

Many of the cells of the body are grouped together to form tissues, structures or organs where they function collectively. These may range from a simple epithelial sheet, which separates one compartment from another, to a complex organ such as the kidney, responsible for removing waste products from the blood and maintaining salt and water homeostasis. The initial

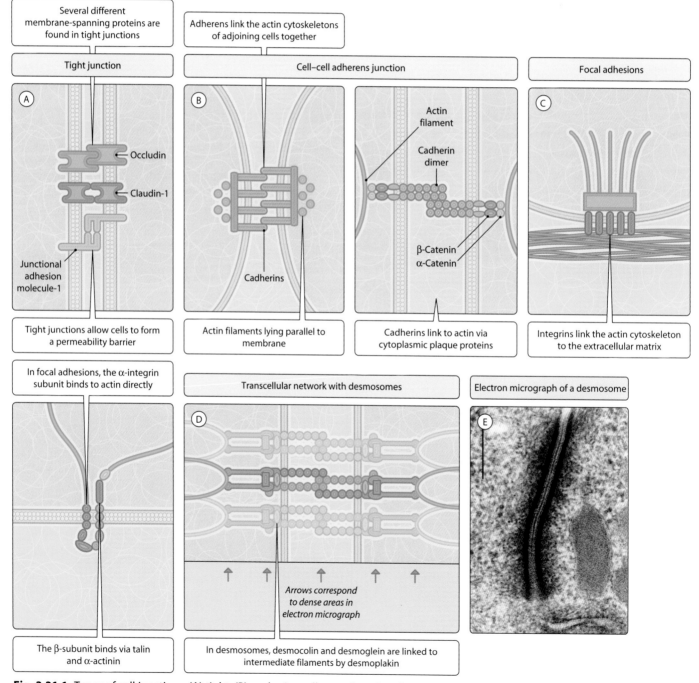

Fig. 3.31.1 Types of cell junctions: (A) tight; (B) anchoring adherens junctions between cells; (C) focal adherens junctions between cells and the matrix; (D) desmosome; (E) EM of a desmosome.

development and subsequent maintenance of these structures requires careful coordination of the growth, replication and death of the cells from which they are made.

Cell–cell and cell–matrix junctions

In order to maintain the structural integrity of tissues and to help individual cells function in an organized and concerted manner, adhesion molecules on one cell link to similar molecules on adjacent cells, or to the extracellular matrix (ECM), forming cellular junctions. There are several types of cell junction (Fig. 3.31.1); tight, anchoring adherens junctions between cells, focal adherens junctions between cells and the ECM, desmosomes, hemi-desmosomes and gap junctions (Ch. 30). Each type performs a different function, and their relative abundance and distribution reflects the type of tissue and the role of the cell within it.

Tight junctions

Tight junctions can be impermeable even to small molecules, a property that allows sheets of epithelial cells to act as permeability barriers. However, tight junctions are not simply fixed structures; the degree of permeability is under physiological control, responding to intracellular signals. For example, solutes leaving the digestive system must traverse a layer of epithelial cells in order to reach the bloodstream, allowing the cells to control which molecules are absorbed. The tight junctions that link these cells also permit the apical and basolateral domains of the plasma membrane, which interface with different physiological compartments, to be separated and prevent their different transporter proteins from mixing.

Anchoring junctions

Anchoring junctions are responsible for maintaining the integrity of tissues. This is achieved by linking the cytoskeletons of adjoining cells to each other, or to the ECM. Adherens junctions contain links to actin and the desmosomes and hemi-desmosomes link to intermediate filaments. All anchoring junctions share a similar basic structure, with the link between membrane-spanning adhesion molecules (cadherin or integrin) and the cytoskeleton being provided by groups of cytoplasmic plaque proteins. The prevalence of anchoring junctions depends on the degree to which a tissue is subjected to mechanical stress.

For example, skin epithelium, which is under constant strain, has large numbers.

Cell–cell adherens junctions

In non-epithelial tissues, cell–cell adherens junctions may be punctate or appear streak-like, but in epithelial tissues they form continuous belts around the entire circumference of each cell. Cells are linked by cadherins, the cytoplasmic domains of which are bound to one of three cytoplasmic plaque proteins (β-catenin, plakoglobin and p120). This complex is linked by α-catenin to the actin filament bundles, which lie parallel to the plasma membrane.

Cell–matrix adherens junctions

In certain cell types, specialized junctions, called focal adhesions, form in specific regions of the plasma membrane where actin bundles terminate. Focal adhesion assembly involves binding of integrins to the ECM, followed by clustering of integrins and binding of cytoplasmic plaque proteins (including talin, vinculin and α-actinin), which provide links to the cytoskeleton.

Desmosomes

Desmosomes link cells and are formed by cadherin-like molecules linked to complexes of cytoplasmic plaque proteins, which act as anchoring sites for intermediate filaments. This provides a strong transcellular network giving the tissue resistance to shear stress.

Hemi-desmosomes

Hemi-desmosomes link cells to the ECM by anchoring the network of intermediate filaments, providing extra strength. They are morphologically similar to desmosomes but the composition of hemi-desmosome plaques is different and the link to the matrix is provided by integrins binding to laminin in the basement membrane.

MUSCULAR DYSTROPHIES

Muscular dystrophies are characterized by progressive muscle weakening and wasting. The most common type, Duchenne muscular dystrophy, is caused by the loss of functional dystrophin, a protein that links the actin cytoskeleton of muscle cells to laminin in the basement membrane via a complex of proteins including α- and β-dystroglycan.

32. The extracellular matrix

Questions
- Are our bodies just collections of cells?
- What are the major constituents of extracellular matrix?
- Are connective tissues merely padding?

Much of the human body comprises connective tissues, which contain few cells. Connective tissues are chiefly made from extracellular matrix (ECM), a mass of specialized proteins and polysaccharides mainly secreted by fibroblasts. It is the ECM that gives conective tissue the ability to resist forces such as shear, tensile force or pressure. Tissues such as skin or bone, which have major structural roles, contain a high proportion of connective tissue.

Collagen and elastin
Members of the collagen family of fibrous proteins are the most abundant proteins in mammals and are major components of skin and bone. Combinations of different α-chain isoforms are wound together in a triple helix to form the different fibrillar and non-fibrillar types of collagen (Fig. 3.32.1). Collagen fibres are laid down in an ordered fashion by fibroblasts, which exert tension on the growing fibre to ensure it lies in the appropriate orientation (relative to the anticipated shearing forces). In bone, sheets of fibrillar collagen are laid down with the fibres of succeeding layers at right angles to the previous one, resulting in considerable strength.

Elastin gives tissues elasticity (Fig. 3.32.2). Elastic fibres are made up of cross-linked elastin monomers and microfibrillar proteins such as fibrillin.

Fibronectin and laminin
Fibronectin is a large disulphide-linked dimeric glycoprotein that plays key roles in cell adhesion and migration in development, malignancy, blood clotting, host defence and in the maintenance of tissue integrity (Fig. 3.32.3).

Laminin is a large glycoprotein in the shape of an asymmetric cross comprising three different disulphide-linked chains. Laminin monomers self-associate to form mesh-like networks, which contribute to the structure of basal laminae (see below). Both fibronectin and laminin are multidomain proteins and are able to bind to several other ECM components and to cell surface receptor proteins including integrins.

Proteoglycans and glycosaminoglycans
Glycosaminoglycans (GAGs) are large polysaccharides (e.g. hyaluronic acid, chondroitin sulphate and heparin). These molecules, which are highly negatively charged making them very hydrophilic, are found as proteoglycans (linked to core proteins). Both GAGs and proteoglycans have several important roles in the body:
- their ability to take up water allows them to occupy large volumes, filling the spaces between cells and providing resistance to compressive forces
- the aqueous gel formed by these molecules acts as a molecular sieve regulating movement of molecules according to size and charge, a property that is important in renal function
- both can bind to extracellular enzymes such as proteinases and to signalling molecules (e.g. growth factors and cytokines).

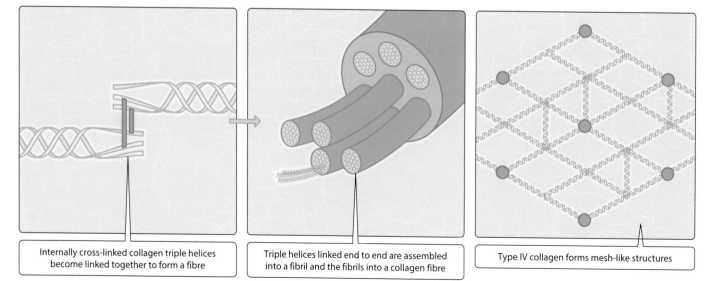

| Internally cross-linked collagen triple helices become linked together to form a fibre | Triple helices linked end to end are assembled into a fibril and the fibrils into a collagen fibre | Type IV collagen forms mesh-like structures |

Fig. 3.32.1 Collagen fibres.

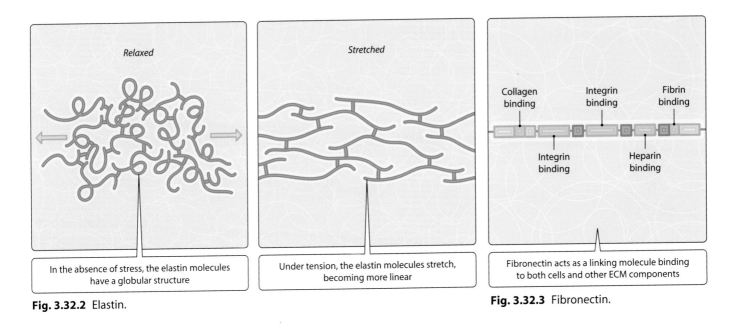

In the absence of stress, the elastin molecules have a globular structure

Under tension, the elastin molecules stretch, becoming more linear

Fibronectin acts as a linking molecule binding to both cells and other ECM components

Fig. 3.32.2 Elastin.

Fig. 3.32.3 Fibronectin.

Basal laminae

In addition to providing tensile strength, elasticity and resistance to compressive forces, ECM components combine to form strong sheets called basal laminae. Basal laminae, which are formed from mesh-like mats of type IV collagen interwoven with other matrix constituents, such as laminin and perlecan, are found in a variety of locations. In the kidney, they play a filtering role, lying between epithelial and endothelial layers in the glomerulus (Fig. 3.32.4). Basal laminae are also found underneath epithelial sheets, where they determine cell polarity and influence cell growth and differentiation, and surrounding muscle cells, where they are vital for the proper organization of neuromuscular junctions.

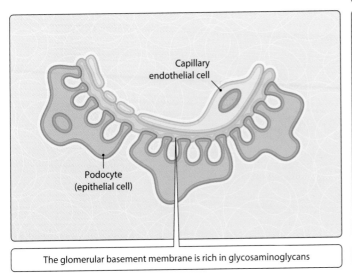

The glomerular basement membrane is rich in glycosaminoglycans

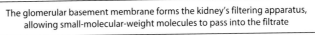
The glomerular basement membrane forms the kidney's filtering apparatus, allowing small-molecular-weight molecules to pass into the filtrate

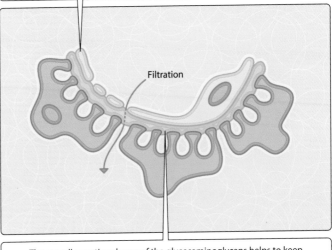

The overall negative charge of the glycosaminoglycans helps to keep proteins in the circulation

Fig. 3.32.4 Basement membranes.

33. Regulation of adhesion

Questions
- How does the extracellular matrix control cell behaviour?
- Are cell junctions always static structures?
- How do adhesion molecules transmit spatial information?

Role of the extracellular matrix

The extracellular matrix (ECM) does not simply provide a protective framework but also has a profound influence on the behaviour of individual cells, imparting spatial information that is crucial for development, differentiation, normal cellular function and resistance to apoptosis. The presence of a basement membrane allows cells to establish and maintain polarity (e.g. in epithelial or endothelial layers). This causes replication to occur within the plane of the cell layer. In addition, any cells that grow into the lumen will have no contact with the ECM and would, therefore, be liable to apoptosis (Fig. 3.33.1).

As well as influencing cells through direct interaction, the ECM also affects them indirectly by controlling the processing, availability and activity of growth factors and proteases. The binding of growth factors to molecules of the ECM prevents them from being dispersed to remote sites and allows local concentrations to reach levels capable of stimulating cellular receptors. ECM components may also provide costimulatory signals, for example through signals activated by integrin binding or as a result of homology to epidermal growth factor (modular proteoglycans). This allows highly localized effects, with different domains of a single molecule playing differing roles simultaneously. The ECM is not a static unchanging modulator of cell behaviour. It is constantly being remodelled by enzymatic breakdown (e.g. by **matrix metalloproteinases**) and synthesis by cells such as **fibroblasts**.

Cell migration is essential not just in development but also in normal growth, wound healing, tissue remodelling and in the immune system. Migration requires the regulated formation and dissolution of adhesive contacts to provide traction for the cell (Ch. 40), but here the emphasis is on cell–matrix rather than cell–cell interactions.

Adhesion molecules as signal transducers

The binding of adhesion molecules to their ligands is not just an isolated event. For example, the avidity with which leukocyte integrins bind to activated vascular endothelium can be modulated by activation of intracellular signalling pathways by chemoattractants or cytokines. Stimulated receptors bind to the intracellular domain of integrins causing a conformational change (the intracellular domains of α- and β-subunits are forced apart causing the extracellular domains to open like a switch-blade) resulting in increased adhesiveness. This process, where a cell's interactions with its extracellular environment respond to an intracellular event, is referred to as inside-out signalling. In addition to allowing the cell to respond to extracellular signals by modulating adhesiveness, integrins also contribute to the intracellular response to extracellular events. Not only does binding of ligand lead to integrin clustering and

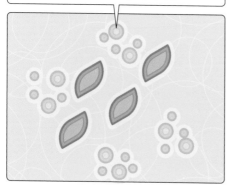

Without attachment, cells fail to proliferate and start to undergo apoptosis

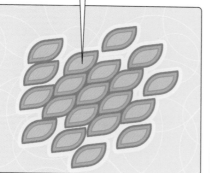

When grown, in the presence of angiogenic growth factors, on cell culture plates coated with collagen (2D), vascular endothelial cells form monolayers with cobblestone-like morphology

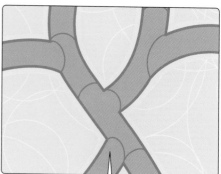

When grown, in the presence of angiogenic growth factors, embedded in a collagen gel (3D), vascular endothelial cells form tube-like structures which resemble capillaries

Fig. 3.33.1 Cells adopt different morphologies in different environments.

focal adhesion assembly, but there is also strong evidence that adhesion molecules have a role in signal transduction in many important cellular processes in addition to those regulating adhesion and migration (Fig. 3.33.2). For example, it has been shown in culture that the mitogenic response of cells, such as fibroblasts, to growth factors is dependent on adhesion to the ECM (anchorage-dependent growth). Integrins and their associated cytoplasmic plaque proteins act as a molecular scaffold bringing signalling molecules together. Adhesion molecule binding also participates in the regulation of the expression of specific genes; for example, the cytoplasmic plaque proteins β-catenin and plakoglobin, when not complexed with cellular junctions, can translocate to the nucleus and interact with certain transcription factors.

DYSREGULATION OF ADHESION IN CANCER

The formation of adherens junctions plays an important role in contact inhibition, where cells stop dividing when they are surrounded by other cells, and anchorage-dependent growth, where cells must be attached to the ECM to avoid death by apoptosis. Loss of the normal adhesive constraints on replication is one of the features of cancer cells (Fig. 3.33.3).

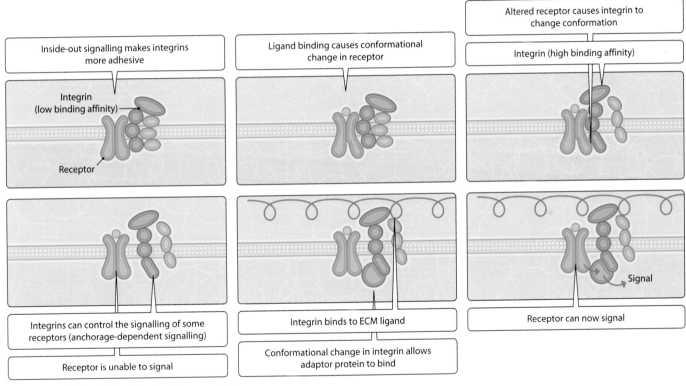

Fig. 3.33.2 Role of integrins in cell responses.

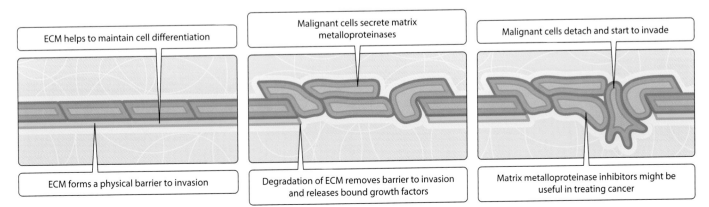

Fig. 3.33.3 Role of matrix metalloproteinases in malignancy.

34. Microfilaments and microtubules: globular cytoskeletal proteins

Questions
- What are the functions of the cytoskeleton?
- How are microfilaments and microtubules assembled?
- Why are tubulin-binding drugs useful in the treatment of cancer?

The cytoskeleton
In eukaryotic cells, the cytoskeleton is a complex and dynamic framework of structural protein filaments that defines the shape of a cell and contributes to changes in cell shape and organelle and cell movement.

Attachment sites
Cellular cytoskeletons are attached to integral proteins in the plasma membrane and through these make attachments to the extracellular matrix (ECM) or adjacent cells (Ch. 31).

Filamentous structures in cytoskeletons
A cell cytoskeleton may contain a combination of three basic filamentous structures: microfilaments (7 nm diameter), intermediate filaments (10 nm) and microtubules (24 nm). Their core structures are formed by actin, intermediate filament proteins and tubulin, respectively. Additional accessory proteins can confer cell-specific and dynamic properties on the cytoskeleton. Accessory proteins can influence the position of the cytoskeleton within the cell by controlling the length of the filamentous structures and their association with other protein complexes, organelles, membranes and the ECM. In addition, they can permit modification of the cytoskeleton in response to intracellular metabolic changes and intracellular signalling pathways, in particular changes in $[Ca^{2+}]_i$. Each of the core structural proteins forms helical filaments, which have a polarity owing to chemically distinct heads and tails. Each protein exists in multiple isoforms, some of which are tissue specific.

Microfilaments
The major constituent of microfilaments is the globular protein actin. Actin filaments (F-actin) consist of two strings of actin monomers (G-actin), which associate with head (+) to tail (−) polarity to form a right-handed helical structure (Fig. 3.34.1). Elongation occurs at both ends but is usually faster at the (+)-end. G-actin contains either bound ATP or bound ADP (Fig. 3.34.2). The rate of binding of G-actin-ATP to growing microfilaments is much faster and binding is followed by rapid ATP hydrolysis, although this is not essential to polymerization. ATP hydrolysis allows a microfilament to treadmill; that is, G-actin-ATP monomers are added at one end while G-actin-ADP dissociates from the other. Growing microfilaments can also break, generating new free ends, which behave as nuclei for further polymerization or may anneal with a second microfilament.

Microtubules
Microtubules are also formed from globular polypeptides. Bidirectional polymerization of αβ-tubulin dimers occurs on small tubulin protofilaments to form the linear polymer (Fig. 3.34.3). Both subunits associate with GTP and GDP and treadmilling may occur at each end of the microtubule associated with GTP hydrolysis. In cells, this is prevented because the slow-growing (−) end is capped by its association with the centrosome complex. Centrosomes comprise a pair of centrioles at right angles to each other, each composed of tubules of nine short triplet microtubules, surrounded by pericentriolar material to which the microtubules are attached.

Microtubules are dynamic structures and rapid depolymerization and repolymerization is a characteristic of their function. New tubulin dimers can be added to rapidly growing protofilaments as long as the terminal tubulin molecule is in the GTP-bound form. If hydrolysis of GTP to GDP occurs in the terminal tubulin, dissociation is favoured and the filament breaks down.

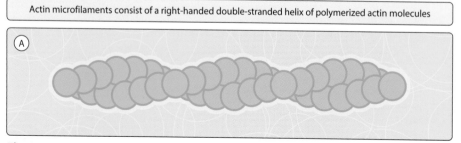

Actin microfilaments consist of a right-handed double-stranded helix of polymerized actin molecules

A

Micrograph of fibroblasts stained to reveal stress fibres in the actin cytoskeletons

B

Fig. 3.34.1 Actin microfilaments.

TUBULIN-BINDING DRUGS IN CANCER THERAPY

Colchicine, nocodazole, taxol and vinblastine all bind to tubulin and interfere with normal tubulin dynamics. Because microtubules are involved in spindle formation in cell division, these drugs are often used as antimitotics in cancer chemotherapy. Colchicine is also used to treat diseases of cell infiltration. In gout, it is used to prevent the migration of neutrophils into joints and it is also used in dermatological diseases that involve leukocyte infiltration (e.g. psoriasis).

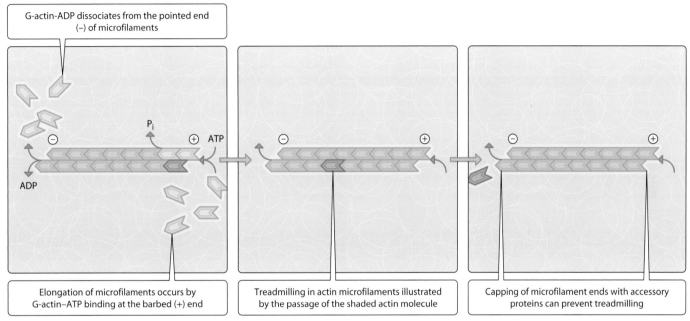

G-actin-ADP dissociates from the pointed end (−) of microfilaments

Elongation of microfilaments occurs by G-actin–ATP binding at the barbed (+) end

Treadmilling in actin microfilaments illustrated by the passage of the shaded actin molecule

Capping of microfilament ends with accessory proteins can prevent treadmilling

Fig. 3.34.2 Treadmilling: movement of G-actin along the microfilament.

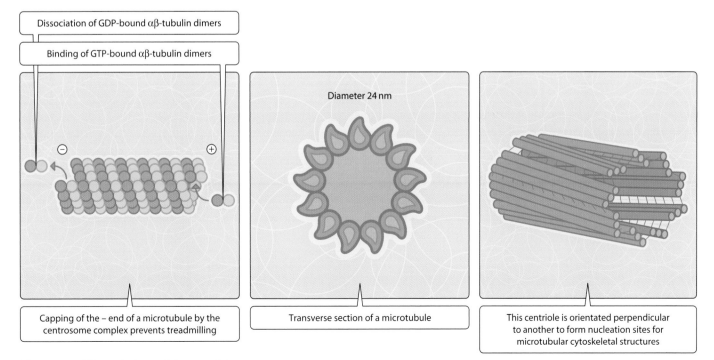

Dissociation of GDP-bound αβ-tubulin dimers

Binding of GTP-bound αβ-tubulin dimers

Diameter 24 nm

Capping of the − end of a microtubule by the centrosome complex prevents treadmilling

Transverse section of a microtubule

This centriole is orientated perpendicular to another to form nucleation sites for microtubular cytoskeletal structures

Fig. 3.34.3 Microtubules and the centriole.

35. Filamentous cytoskeletal proteins

Questions
- How are intermediate filaments assembled?
- What are the major components of the erythrocyte cytoskeleton?
- What is the molecular basis of the haemolytic anaemia hereditary spherocytosis?

Intermediate filaments

Unlike actin and tubulin, which are globular proteins, the intermediate filament proteins are fibrous and are a much more heterogeneous group of proteins. They form cytoplasmic filamentous structures that are intermediate in diameter (10 nm) between microfilaments and microtubules (Fig. 3.35.1). Each type of filament is composed of a defined protein or combination of proteins. Each intermediate filament protein has a homologous α-helical core structure with subunit-specific N- and C-termini of variable length. Filament formation is initiated by the formation of a parallel, coiled-coil structure composed of the homologous core structure of two subunits.

Intermediate filaments are then formed by polymerization of these dimeric structures. Being based on a homologous core structure, copolymerization of mixed intermediate filament oligomers is possible when certain subunits are coexpressed in the same tissue. Not all subunit combinations are stable. Where coexpression of incompatible subunits occurs, homo-oligomers of each protein are formed (e.g. keratins and vimentin in epithelial cells).

Spectrin–actin cytoskeleton of the erythrocyte

The best understood cytoskeleton is the spectrin–actin cytoskeleton of erythrocytes, which confers the biconcave shape to these cells (Fig. 3.35.2). This cytoskeleton is based on the peripheral membrane protein spectrin, which is a long, rod-like molecule consisting of α- and β-subunits that wind together to form a heterodimer. Heterodimers form a head-to-head association to form heterotetramers of $\alpha_2\beta_2$ and these are cross-linked into networks by short actin protofilaments ($\approx$ 14 actin monomers), which associate towards the ends of the spectrin heterotetramers. This interaction is stabilized by a protein called

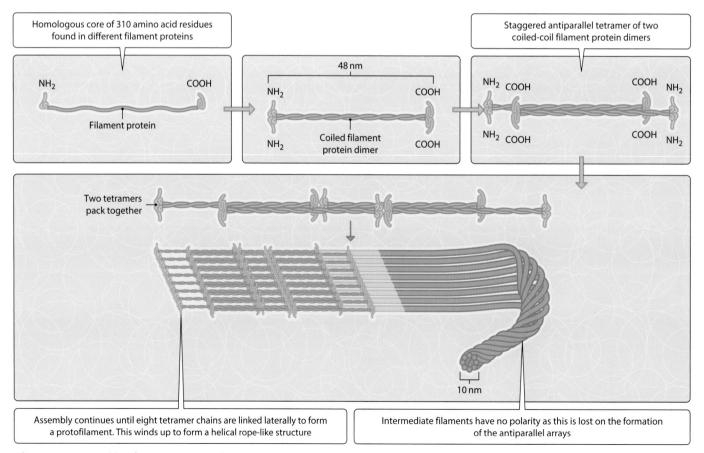

Homologous core of 310 amino acid residues found in different filament proteins

NH₂   COOH

Filament protein

48 nm

NH₂   COOH

NH₂   COOH

Coiled filament protein dimer

Staggered antiparallel tetramer of two coiled-coil filament protein dimers

NH₂ COOH   COOH NH₂

NH₂ COOH   COOH NH₂

Two tetramers pack together

10 nm

Assembly continues until eight tetramer chains are linked laterally to form a protofilament. This winds up to form a helical rope-like structure

Intermediate filaments have no polarity as this is lost on the formation of the antiparallel arrays

Fig. 3.35.1 Assembly of an intermediate filament.

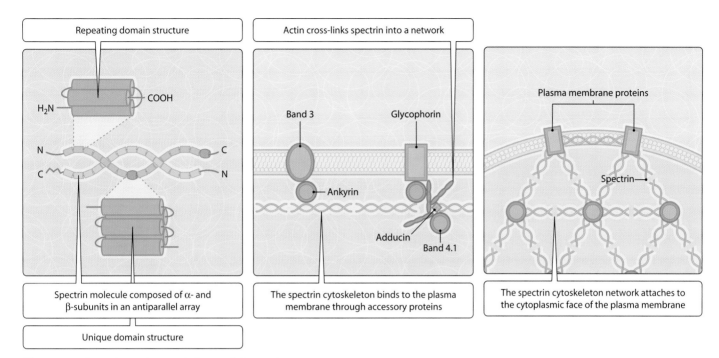

Fig. 3.35.2 Spectrin–actin cytoskeleton of the erythrocyte.

band 4.1 (after its relative migration in electrophoresis) and adducin. The spectrin–actin network is attached to the plasma membrane through accessory proteins that link spectrin to integral membrane proteins. Ankyrin (band 4.9) forms a link between the spectrin and the anion exchange protein (band 3), and band 4.1 forms an association with glycophorin A. Attachment of integral membrane proteins to the cytoskeleton in this way restricts the lateral mobility of membrane proteins and is one mechanism by which membrane proteins may be anchored in different tissues.

Spectrin supergene family

Spectrin or spectrin-like molecules are also found in non-erythroid tissues where they contribute to cytoskeletal structures close to the plasma membrane but also as multifunctional cross-linkers within the cytoplasm. The α-subunit of spectrin may associate with an alternatively spliced erythroid β-subunit or with a non-erythroid spectrin β-subunit to produce fodrin (spectrin II).

Two other proteins with spectrin-like repeating structures of three α-helices and conserved N-terminal domains are α-actinin and dystrophin. Alpha-actinin is an actin-bundling protein (see Z discs; Ch. 36) and dystrophin is proposed to attach actin filaments to the plasma membrane in skeletal muscle.

 HAEMOLYTIC ANAEMIAS

The erythrocyte cytoskeleton is important in maintaining the deformability necessary for erythrocytes to make their passage through capillary beds without lysis. In the common dominant form of hereditary spherocytosis, spectrin levels may be depleted by 40–50%. The cells round up and become much less resistant to lysis and are cleared by capillaries in the spleen. The shortened in vivo survival of red blood cells and the inability of the bone marrow to compensate for their reduced lifespan leads to haemolytic anaemia. Similarly, in hereditary elliptocytosis, a common defect is a spectrin molecule that is unable to form heterotetramers, resulting in fragile ellipsoid cells. Even simple treatment with cytochalasin drugs, which cap the growing end of polymerizing actin filaments, can alter the deformability of the erythrocyte.

 CYTOSKELETON AND BLOOD PRESSURE

Mutations affecting the cytoskeletal linker protein adducin have been shown to be associated genetically with essential hypertension. These mutants modify membrane ion transport in a way that is similar to perturbations seen in hypertensive patients. It may be that cytoskeletal perturbation resulting in altered ion homeostasis in vascular tissues may contribute to the development of hypertension in some patients.

36. Skeletal muscle contraction

Questions
- What is the structure of the thick and thin filaments of contractile tissues?
- To what do the 'A band', 'I band' and 'Z line' relate in the sarcomere?
- How is the energy of ATP hydrolysis coupled to movement in actomyosin?

Microfilamentous structure of skeletal muscle

In contractile cells, the cytoskeleton is modified to provide the contractile machinery. Shortening in muscle cells is mediated by the progressive overlap of interdigitated thick and thin filaments.

Thick filaments

The core of thick filaments is formed from myosin (Fig. 3.36.1). Myosin molecules are composed of two myosin heavy chains, intertwined to form a rigid tail structure with two head regions at one end. The head regions interact with two light chains each and provide a site for interaction with polymerized actin filaments and a catalytic ATPase domain. Thick filaments are formed by the tail-to-tail association of myosin molecules to form insoluble, rod-like complexes of between 300 and 400 molecules. The head groups protrude to the outside of the structure at both ends and are aligned for optimal interaction with adjacent actin filaments, leaving a central bare zone.

Thin filaments

Thin filaments are stable structures composed of F-actin microfilaments, tropomyosin and troponin. Tropomyosin is a long rod-like molecule; at rest, it lies along the surface of the helical structure of thin filaments blocking the interaction with

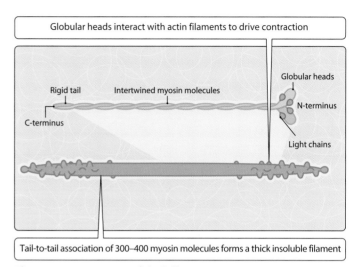

Fig. 3.36.1 Formation of thick filaments.

thick myosin filaments. In response to raised $[Ca^{2+}]_i$, tropomyosin moves to the groove region, revealing the myosin-binding sites and permitting activity of the contractile machinery (Fig. 3.36.2). Calcium is, therefore, the trigger for and facilitator of muscle contraction by controlling the allosteric inhibition of thin and thick filament interaction. Sensitivity to Ca^{2+} is conferred by troponin.

The sarcomere

Vertebrate skeletal muscle has a striated appearance and is made up of parallel, multinucleated cells containing bundles of myofibrils. In relaxed muscle, the contractile element has a repeating structure (2.4 μm): an alternating pattern of light (I band, isotropic) and dark (A band, anisotropic) bands. A dark line bisecting the I band is the Z band (Z disc) and the segment

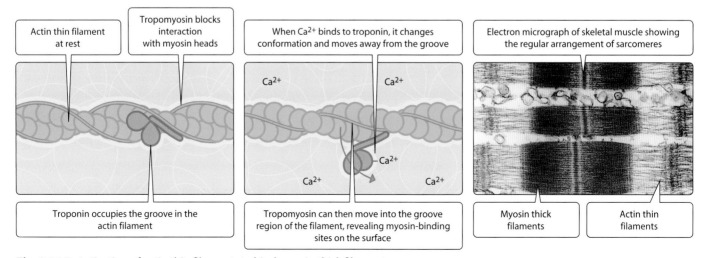

Fig. 3.36.2 Activation of actin thin filaments to bind myosin thick filaments.

of myofibril between two Z discs is defined as a sarcomere (Fig. 3.36.3). Thin filaments are attached to Z discs and constitute the light half I band and the darker region of the A band at each end of the sarcomere. The A band represents the distribution of myosin thick filaments. On muscle contraction, the distance between Z discs is reduced (from 2.4 µm to ≈ 1.6 µm) as is the length of the I band. The length of the A band remains unchanged. This important observation forms the basis of the 'sliding filament' model of muscle contraction.

The sliding filament model of muscle contraction: role of ATP

The opposite movement of thick and thin filaments during contraction is achieved by a cyclic interaction between actin and myosin of attachment, pulling and detachment driven by the myosin head groups (Fig. 3.36.4). At rest, the myosin head groups contain ADP and P_i in their catalytic site. On binding actin, P_i is released, and the head undergoes a large rotation in the 'hinge' region of the molecule between the head group and tail. This large conformational change, known as the 'powerstroke', pulls the myosin molecule along the actin filament by approximately 7.5 nm. At the end of the powerstroke, ADP is released from the myosin active site and is replaced by ATP. This leads to a rapid dissociation of the myosin heads from actin and reversal of the conformational change of the head group. Hydrolysis of the bound ATP returns the myosin head group to the high-energy, myosin-ADP-P_i form, priming it for a further round of the cycle. The myosin head groups in thick filaments do not move in synchrony but rather can be found at different phases at any one moment, ensuring smooth contraction overall.

RIGOR MORTIS

In the absence of ATP, the actin–myosin interaction at the end of the power stroke remains associated in the so-called rigor complex. This is the process of rigor mortis in dead muscle.

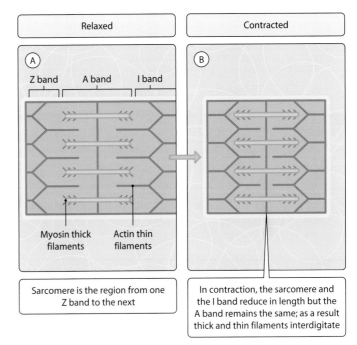

| Relaxed | Contracted |

Sarcomere is the region from one Z band to the next

In contraction, the sarcomere and the I band reduce in length but the A band remains the same; as a result thick and thin filaments interdigitate

Fig. 3.36.3 The sarcomere.

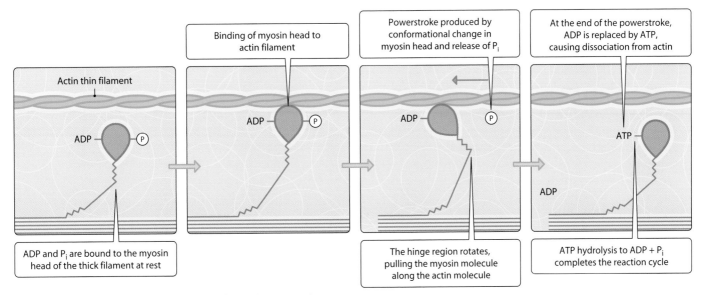

Binding of myosin head to actin filament

Powerstroke produced by conformational change in myosin head and release of P_i

At the end of the powerstroke, ADP is replaced by ATP, causing dissociation from actin

Actin thin filament

ADP and P_i are bound to the myosin head of the thick filament at rest

The hinge region rotates, pulling the myosin molecule along the actin molecule

ATP hydrolysis to ADP + P_i completes the reaction cycle

Fig. 3.36.4 The 'sliding filament' model of muscle contraction.

37. Excitation–contraction coupling in skeletal, cardiac and smooth muscle

Questions
- How is electrical excitation translated into a contractile event in skeletal muscle?
- How does this process differ in cardiac and smooth muscle types?
- How is the arrangement of contractile fibres in smooth muscle different to that in skeletal and cardiac muscles?

Skeletal muscle
In skeletal muscle, the Ca^{2+} for contraction comes from the sarcoplasmic reticulum (SR) Ca^{2+} stores. At the A–I band junction, a regular structure of tubules, known as a triad, is formed that consists of two SR tubules, called terminal cisternae, separated by a deep invagination of the plasma membrane, called a transverse tubule or t-tubule. The release of Ca^{2+} is triggered by electrical activity in the sarcolemma (muscle plasma membrane) (Fig. 3.37.1C).

The t-tubular system ensures that the action potential stimulus for contraction is transmitted rapidly deep within the fibre. The L-type voltage-sensitive Ca^{2+} channels in the t-tubule system change conformation in response to the depolarization but, rather than admit Ca^{2+} to the myocyte, these channels are physically coupled to ryanodine-sensitive Ca^{2+} channels in the SR and stimulate these to open and release Ca^{2+} from the SR store directly over the sarcomere structures that will initiate contraction. The Ca^{2+} in the cytoplasm is returned to the SR via Ca^{2+}-ATPase proteins in the SR membrane.

Cardiac muscle
Cardiac muscle is composed of rectangular, mononucleated muscle cells that have a striated appearance. The cardiac-specific contractile elements are organized into sarcomeres, similar to those in skeletal muscle (Fig. 3.37.1A). Cardiac cells interdigitate such that intercalated disc structures form irregular junctions between transverse and longitudinal aspects of adjacent cells. Junctional complexes within the intercalated disc structures between cardiac cells provide attachment sites for thin filaments at the sarcolemma and effectively connect the thin filaments of adjacent cells, performing a similar function to Z bands in skeletal muscle. In the longitudinal aspect of intercalated discs, gap junctions form. These junctions are permeable to small solutes and ions. By allowing communication between the cytoplasm of adjacent cells, these structures result in electrical coupling and, thereby, a synchronous contractile response.

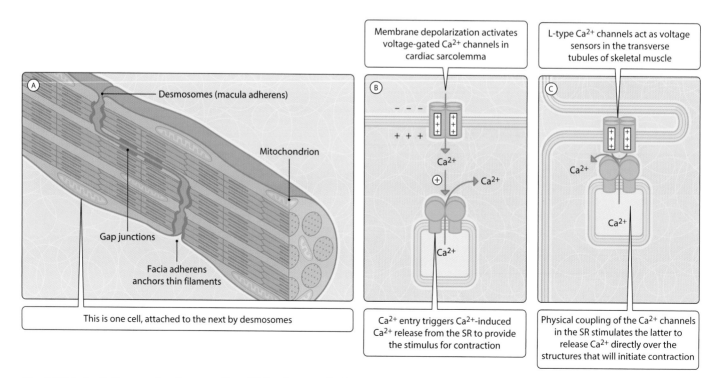

Fig. 3.37.1 Excitation–contraction coupling. (A) Cardiac muscle; (B) coupling in cardiac muscle; (C) coupling in skeletal muscle.

The majority of the Ca^{2+} required to initiate contraction comes from the SR. In this case, on myocyte depolarization, Ca^{2+} entering through L-type voltage-gated Ca^{2+} channels triggers release of stored Ca^{2+} by Ca^{2+}-induced Ca^{2+} release (CICR; Fig. 3.17.1B); this is in contrast to the physical coupling to SR Ca^{2+} channels in skeletal muscle.

Smooth muscle

Smooth muscle is composed of elongated, tapering, mono-nucleated cells linked by structural junctional contacts and gap junctions. The actomyosin sliding filament complexes are less organized than in striated muscle, do not form sarcomeres and do not appear striated. In this tissue, the actomyosin filaments are interconnected by dense bodies and they are connected to the sarcolemma by intermediate filaments. Smooth muscle isoforms of actin and myosin produce slower contraction than skeletal muscle but more sustained tension.

In smooth muscle, most of the Ca^{2+} to initiate contraction is derived from outside the cell (Fig. 3.37.2). Troponin is absent in smooth muscle. Instead, Ca^{2+} sensitivity is mediated by calmodulin, which binds and activates myosin light chain kinase (MLCK), leading to phosphorylation of myosin light chains.

Smooth muscle myosin head groups bind actin filaments only when the light chains are in the phosphorylated form. On restoration of resting $[Ca^{2+}]_i$, the calmodulin dissociates from the MLCK rendering it inactive. Relaxation of smooth muscle follows when a myosin light chain phosphatase returns the myosin molecule to the inactive form. The force of contraction of smooth muscle can be regulated by other signaling pathways to give a more relaxed state (Fig. 3.37.3).

MALIGNANT HYPERTHERMIA

Malignant hyperthermia is a rare, congential condition that is associated with a perturbation of excitation–contraction coupling in skeletal muscle. It is induced by neuromuscular-blocking drugs (e.g. suxamethonium (succinylcholine)) and volatile anaesthetics (e.g. halothane), which produce increases in $[Ca^{2+}]_i$ and skeletal muscle metabolism. Clinically, this results in intense muscle spasm and a rapid rise in body temperature and can be potentially fatal. Treatment is with dantrolene, which inhibits skeletal muscle contraction by inhibiting CICR from the SR. Although the cause of malignant hyperthermia is unknown, mutations in the ryanodine-sensitive Ca^{2+} channel responsible for CICR have been identified in affected patients.

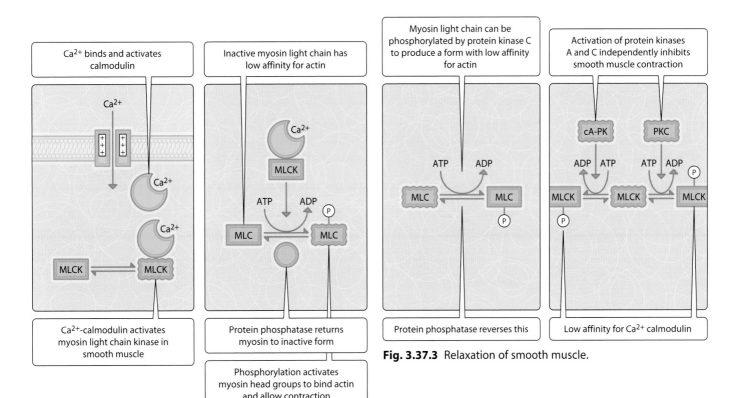

Fig. 3.37.3 Relaxation of smooth muscle.

Fig. 3.37.2 Excitation–contraction coupling in smooth muscle.

38. Microtubules in vesicular and organelle transport

Questions
- How is directional trafficking of intracellular vesicles achieved?
- How is vesicle trafficking driven?
- How may disruption of microtubular structures result in neurodegeneration?

Transport of organelles and membrane-bound vesicles in eukaryotic cells is directed along 'tracks' of single microtubules by a 'walking' mechanism (Fig. 3.38.1). The molecular motors for this movement are myosin-like ATPases, kinesin and dynein. Kinesin drives movement from the (−)-end (centrosome) of the microtubule to the (+)-end while cytoplasmic dynein drives movement in the opposite direction. Since microtubules are usually arranged with their centromeres near the centre of the cell, kinesin drives anterograde movement from the centre to the periphery, while dynein drives retrograde movement towards the centre. The ATP-dependent attachment of kinesin or dynein head groups to the microtubule drives the movement of the vesicle along the microtubule at up to 5 μm/s.

Kinesin and dynein
Kinesin is a large elongated multisubunit protein. At one end, two globular head regions provide the sites for ATP hydrolysis and cross-bridge formation to tubulin. The other flattened end interacts with proteins in the transported vesicle, attaching the vesicle to the microtubular track (Fig. 3.38.2). Unlike myosin and dynein, which release bound protein when ATP binds, the interaction of ATP with the kinesin head group promotes binding to the microtubule. Hydrolysis of the ATP molecule occurs while the microtubule is bound, causing the release of the crossbridge and a step along the microtubule. This results in a 'hand-over-hand' movement along the microtubule. There is considerable similarity between the structures of the kinesin and dynein head groups and the kinetics of ATP hydrolysis catalysed by the two molecules. The direction of movement of the two molecules along the microtubule may simply reflect whether the molecule walks 'forwards' or 'backwards' during the reaction cycle.

Axonal transport in neurons
Directional transport along microtubules is particularly important in the axons of neurons, where cellular materials may need to be transported over relatively large distances (Fig. 3.38.3). Kinesin drives the fast anterograde movement of vesicles containing synaptic plasma membrane components, synaptic vesicles containing neurotransmitters and mitochondria towards the nerve terminal. Fast retrograde transport of endocytic vesicles and mitochondria is driven by dynein. In addition, axonal microtubules direct the slow unidirectional axonal transport in the anterograde direction of cytoskeletal elements such as actin, actin-binding proteins, fodrin, clathrin and cytoplasmic enzymes, and the even slower transport of cytoplasmic components such as preassembled networks of neurofilaments, microtubules and associated proteins.

⊕ MOTOR NEURON DISEASES

Motor neuron diseases are characterized by progressive muscle weakness and atrophy. Defective axonal transport has been suggested to contribute to neuronal degeneration in this group of conditions. Consistent with this hypothesis, a mutation in the large subunit of the protein dynactin has been identified recently in a family with inherited progressive motor neuron disease. Dynactin is a linker between dynein, microtubules and the cargo. The mutation results in reduced microtubule binding.

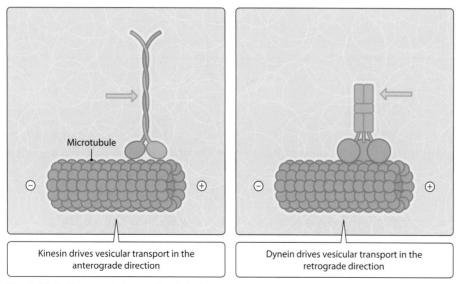

Kinesin drives vesicular transport in the anterograde direction	Dynein drives vesicular transport in the retrograde direction

Fig. 3.38.1 Transport along microtubules.

ALZHEIMER'S DISEASE

Alzheimer's disease is a neurodegenerative condition associated with the deposition of β-amyloid plaques and neurofibrillary tangles. In normal cells, the microtubule-associated protein Tau is important in stabilizing microtubular tracks and, therefore, plays a key role in the maintenance of axonal transport. In Alzheimer's disease, for reasons that are unknown, Tau protein becomes abnormally heavily phosphorylated. This causes it to form paired helical filaments, which are deposited as neurofibrillary tangles, resulting in impairment of axonal transport. The loss of efficient axonal transport reduces neurotransmitter release from neurons and probably explains the decrease in cognitive ability in patients with this disease.

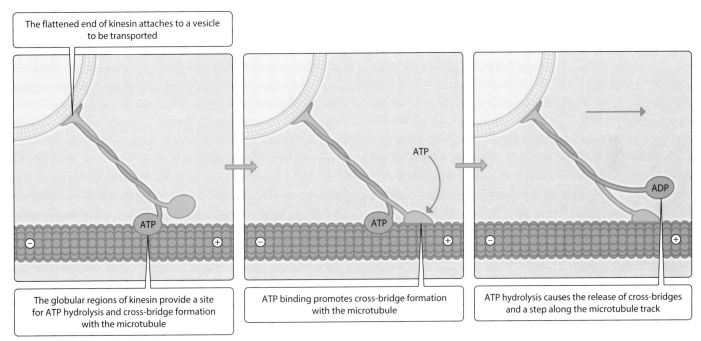

The flattened end of kinesin attaches to a vesicle to be transported

The globular regions of kinesin provide a site for ATP hydrolysis and cross-bridge formation with the microtubule

ATP binding promotes cross-bridge formation with the microtubule

ATP hydrolysis causes the release of cross-bridges and a step along the microtubule track

Fig. 3.38.2 Role of kinesin in vesicle transport.

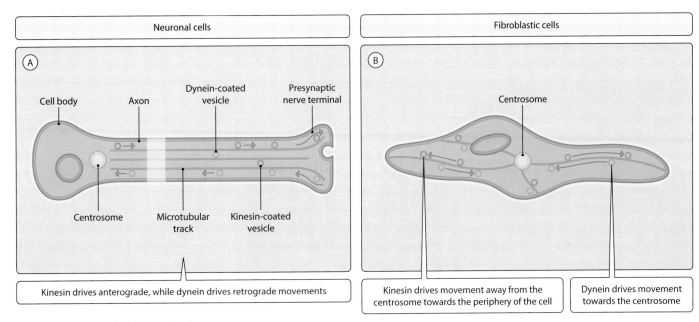

Neuronal cells

Fibroblastic cells

A

Cell body   Axon   Dynein-coated vesicle   Presynaptic nerve terminal

Centrosome   Microtubular track   Kinesin-coated vesicle

B

Centrosome

Kinesin drives anterograde, while dynein drives retrograde movements

Kinesin drives movement away from the centrosome towards the periphery of the cell

Dynein drives movement towards the centrosome

Fig. 3.38.3 Microtubules in vesicular transport.

39. Microfilamentous structures in non-muscle cells

Questions
- What roles may actomyosin structures have in non-muscle cells?
- What are the differences in structure and function of cilia and flagella?
- What may be the physiological consequences of immotile cilia syndrome?

Actomyosin structures

In addition to muscle tissues, microfilamentous actomyosin structures are also found in non-muscle cells where contractile properties are required. For example, actomyosin contributes to intracellular stress fibres, to the flattening of attached cells in cell culture and in cellular locomotion (Ch. 40). Actomyosin structures are also important during telophase in the cell cycle to form the contractile ring that begins cell division (Ch. 44).

Unlike striated muscle, the contractile apparatus in non-muscle cells is constantly dissociating and reforming depending on the state of stimulation of the cell. In the inactive, dephosphorylated form, the myosin molecule takes up an independent globular form. On phosphorylation of the myosin light chain by myosin light chain kinase, the myosin molecule extends to its rod-like form, releasing the tail domain to form bipolar thick filaments and the head domain to form cross-bridges with thin filament actin.

Microvilli

To increase the surface area of epithelial tissues, the apical membrane is folded into numerous finger-like projections called microvilli (Fig. 3.39.1). Microvilli are packed with bundles of actin filaments; these are cross-linked to maintain their shape and are attached to the tip of each microvillus by the growing (+)-end. Calmodulin and a myosin-like, actin-stimulated ATPase link the actin filaments to the inner surface of the plasma membrane. Where the actin bundles protrude into the cell, they interact with a complex cytoplasmic meshwork structure called the terminal web. This structure is linked via fodrin to the cytoskeleton of intermediate filaments.

Cilia and flagella

Cilia and flagella are specialized surface appendages of cells that have a beating function. Cilia are found grouped in ciliary fields in tissues such as pulmonary and oviduct epithelia. Synchronous beating of cilia in waves across the pulmonary epithelium permits the removal of particles from the lungs, and in the oviduct ciliary beating aids the progress of the ovum down the Fallopian tube (Fig. 3.39.2). Cilia are usually approximately

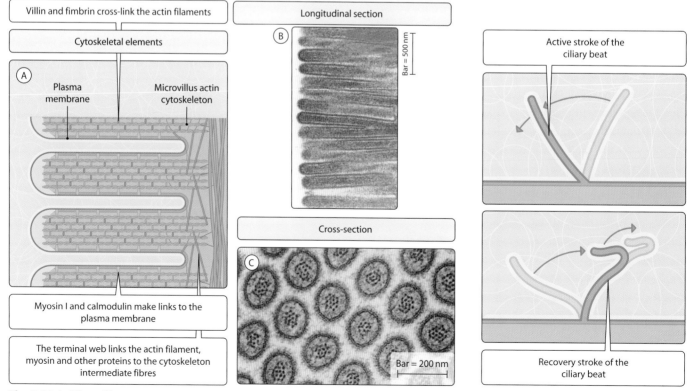

Fig. 3.39.1 Microvillus structure.

Fig. 3.39.2 The ciliary beat.

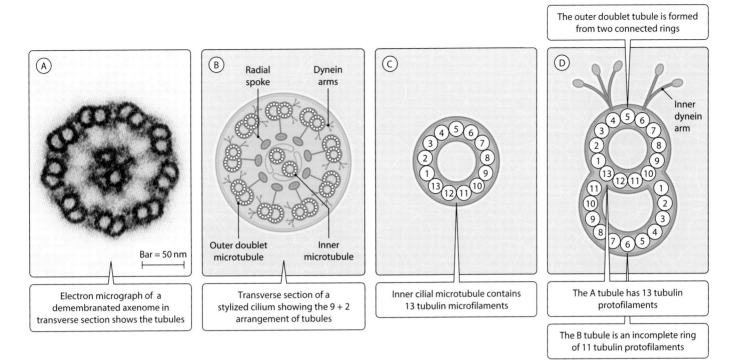

Fig. 3.39.3 Arrangement of tubules in a cilium.

10 μm in length but they can extend up to 200 μm in some cells. In contrast, the flagellum is a long single motile element that provides a swimming mechanism. This structure is of primary importance in the swimming of spermatozoa.

Axonemal structure of cilia and flagella

Both cilia and flagella share a similar axoneme nine-plus-two structure based on tubulin microtubules (Fig. 3.39.3). These stable microtubular structures, which extend the length of the cilium or flagellum, form an array of two central tubules surrounded by nine circumferential doublet tubules linked to the central tubules via radial spoke proteins. Emanating from the A tubule of the microtubule doublets are inner and outer dynein arms. When ATP binds, the dynein head groups detach from the B tubule and reattach further along the tubule. On ATP hydrolysis, the dynein molecule returns to its resting conformation, which produces a sliding force between the two adjacent tubules. The radial spokes restrict longitudinal movement and this produces a bend in the axoneme structure (Fig. 3.39.4). This mechanism must be tightly regulated so that activity occurs only in part of the structure at any one time to produce a beating motion.

Bacterial flagella

The structure of a bacterial flagellum is much simpler than the eukaryotic structure; it consists of a filament of a single protein that is rotated by a basal body structure at the level of the membrane. This rotation produces the characteristic spiralling motion of a moving bacterium.

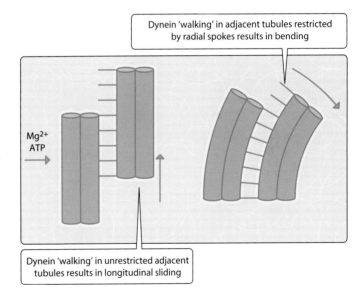

Fig. 3.39.4 Production of bending in a cilium.

 ANAESTHETIC DEPRESSION OF CILIARY MOVEMENT

The carpet of mucus that coats the bronchioles of the lung, trapping inhaled particles and bacteria, is normally propelled out of the lungs by ciliary beating. Anaesthetics may interfere with this by depressing ciliary motility; this increases the risk of mucous accumulation and infection in the lung.

40. Cell migration/motility

Questions
- How do cells initiate movement?
- What is the driving force for cell movement?
- How can directional cell locomotion be specified?
- Why do plasma membrane components move away from the direction of cellular movement?

Cell locomotion is important for many processes: immunological tissue infiltration in inflammation and immunity, fertilization, embryological development, and tissue repair and turnover. The internal mechanisms can propel extracellular materials past cells in processes such as wound healing. Three types of cell motion can be described: random motion; chemokinesis, a non-directional increase in cell movement in response to a chemical stimulus; and chemotaxis, the purposeful movement towards or away from a chemical stimulus.

Cilia and flagella in cell motility
Single cells such as spermatozoa move by beating of a flagellum or cilia. In tissues such as epithelia, cilia assist in the passage of extracellular materials past the cells (e.g. for removal of mucus and debris from the lungs).

Cell movements over the substratum
Cells may crawl over their substratum in a jerky movement by about a millimetre or so a day (Fig. 3.40.1) using focal adhesions to attach forward-directed protrusions to the substrate. In cell culture, the dorsal surface of flattened fibroblasts becomes characteristically 'ruffled' at and behind the leading edge; this reflects sites of rapid actin polymerization moving backwards away from the leading edge (Fig. 3.40.2). Ruffling may simply reflect a lack of adhesion to this cell surface. Similar retrograde

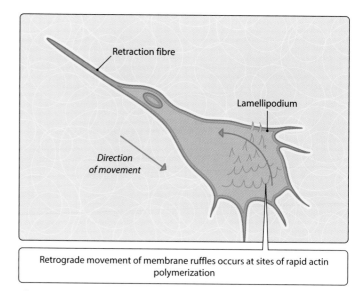

Retrograde movement of membrane ruffles occurs at sites of rapid actin polymerization

Fig. 3.40.2 Formation of 'ruffles' in a migrating fibroblast.

movement of structures on the 'ventral' surface may provide the backwards driving or tractive force for movement of the leading edge.

Paradoxically, as the cell moves forwards there is a retrograde movement of larger membrane constituents away from the leading edge. A 'raking' mechanism has been proposed in which larger molecules associate with transmembranous adhesion proteins that, in turn, are linked to backward-moving actin microfilaments in the advancing tip of the lamellipodium (Fig. 3.40.3). The microfilaments have their growing ends towards the leading edge such that treadmilling of the filaments results in extension of the lamellipodium forwards and retrograde motion of the adhesion proteins. Inhibition of actin filament polymerization at the growing end by proximity of the lamellipodial membrane may be prevented simply by thermal

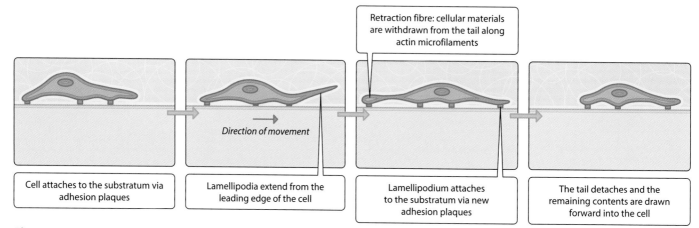

Retraction fibre: cellular materials are withdrawn from the tail along actin microfilaments

Direction of movement

Cell attaches to the substratum via adhesion plaques

Lamellipodia extend from the leading edge of the cell

Lamellipodium attaches to the substratum via new adhesion plaques

The tail detaches and the remaining contents are drawn forward into the cell

Fig. 3.40.1 Fibroblast locomotion over a substratum.

motion of the filament end or by osmotic swelling at the leading edge, providing space for continued polymerization. Fungal cytochalasins, which bind to the growing (+)-end of actin filaments and block polymerization, also block cell locomotion.

To restore membrane macromolecules and lipids removed by the raking activity, vesicles derived from the Golgi apparatus fuse with the lamellipodial membrane, reincorporating new and recycled molecules at the leading edge. In some, but not all, cells, vesicles from the Golgi apparatus are directed by microtubules. Even before lamellipodia are formed, the microtubule-organizing centre (MTOC) is orientated such that the vesicles

from the Golgi are directed to the leading edge, thereby polarizing the cell. The direction of chemotactic cell migration is determined by membrane receptors for chemotactic stimuli. How these messages are translated into intracellular events remains unknown. As the cell moves forwards, actin filaments depolymerize and cellular materials are withdrawn from the tail of the cell along receding actin microfilaments. This results in cell narrowing to form retraction fibres. Ultimately, the tail detaches and is drawn forward into the cell. Proteases secreted near focal adhesions also contribute to detachment of trailing regions (e.g. urokinase).

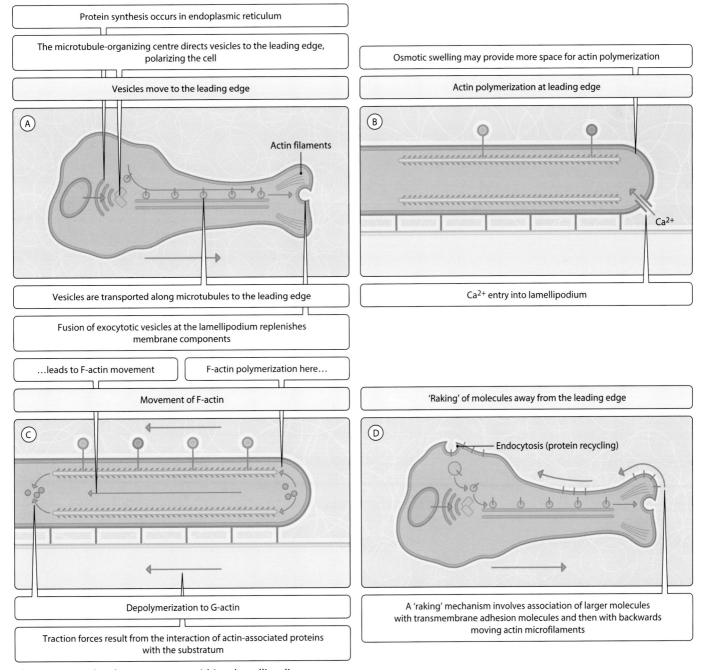

Fig. 3.40.3 Molecular movements within a lamellipodium.

41. The cell cycle

Questions
- How is the chromosome complement of daughter cells maintained during cell division of somatic cells?
- How is cell division regulated?
- What is the role of the cytoskeleton in cell division?

Cell division is important for growth, development, repair and replacement of dead cells. In an organism with multiple cell types and tissues, cell proliferation must be tightly regulated: loss of control is cancer.

Stages of the cell cycle
The process of cell division is cyclical and unidirectional (Fig. 3.41.1). The period between successive cell divisions is termed the interphase. Interphase begins with a period of rapid biosynthesis and cell growth, G_1 (gap) phase, to provide sufficient cellular constituents for two daughter cells. This phase is the most variable in duration (minutes to months). In non-dividing tissues, cells withdraw from the cell cycle into a resting state (G_0) but can re-enter G_1 upon stimulation. After G_1, the cell moves into S phase, when the complete genomic DNA is duplicated. A second gap phase, G_2, then prepares the cell for the M phase, where mitosis, the division of nuclear material, and cytokinesis, the process of cytoplasmic division, occur such that the two daughter cells each receive a complete copy of the genomic DNA.

Proliferation of quiescent cells (mitogenesis)
Proliferation of quiescent cells (transition from G_0 to G_1) can be induced by mitogens, leading to the expression of responsive

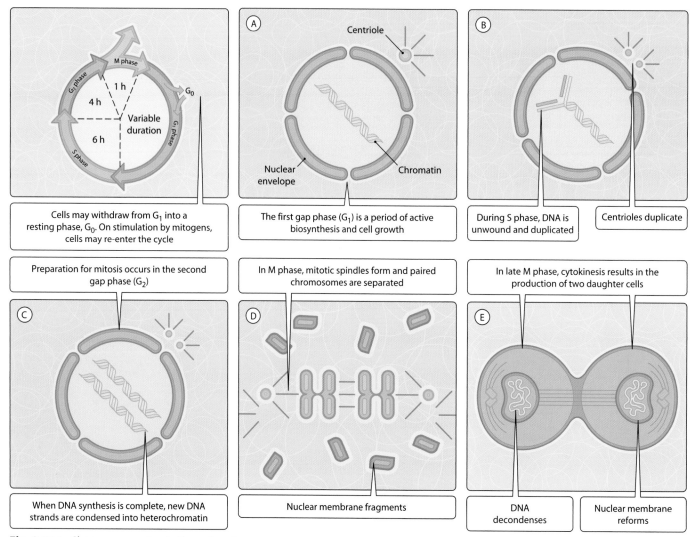

Fig. 3.41.1 Changes occurring in the cell cycle.

genes and progression of the cell through G_1 phase and past a 'restriction point' (mammalian cells) or START (yeast). Once past the restriction point, cells become committed to a complete division cycle, no longer require the presence of growth factors and are unresponsive to antimitogenic signals.

Regulation of the cell cycle

Progression is controlled at 'checkpoints' between the stages (e.g. restriction point, mitosis entry and mitosis exit) (Fig. 3.41.2). These monitor, respectively, the availability of nutrients/growth factors, DNA replication/damage and assembly of the mitotic spindle. Transition between stages is triggered by increased activity of specific cyclin-dependent protein kinases (CDK) (Fig. 3.41.2B). Each CDK phosphorylates, and thereby modulates, the activity of a subset of target proteins specific for progression through individual transitions within the cell cycle.

Control of cyclin-dependent protein kinase activity by cyclin expression

Levels of CDK proteins remain relatively constant throughout the cell cycle but their activity is regulated at different stages. The CDKs are activated primarily by the binding of specific cyclins. The levels of the different cyclins rise and fall at different points in the cell cycle and thus produce temporal activation of their specific CDK. For example, the synthesis of cyclin B is rela-

tively constant and concentrations rise in a linear manner until a threshold is reached when Cdc2 is activated and the cell proceeds into mitosis. At mitosis, the rate of cyclin B breakdown is accelerated and the stimulation of Cdc2 is terminated.

CDKs are also subject to complex modulation in response to several intracellular signalling pathways. This serves to integrate intra- and extracellular signals reflecting nutritional status and intercellular communication.

Tumour suppressor genes regulate the passage into S phase

Substrates for CDKs are still being characterized. However, one mechanism at the G_1–S checkpoint may involve the hyper-phosphorylation of negative cell cycle regulators, such as the retinoblastoma tumour suppressor gene product (pRb), to overcome their suppression of passage from G_1 (Fig. 3.41.2C). In normal quiescent cells and early G_1, pRb is found in a hypophosphorylated form, which actively binds several cytoplasmic proteins. Phosphorylation of pRb by G_1 CDK (CDK2/cyclin D) results in the release of these proteins, including transcription factors of the E2F family, which go on to activate transcription of the S-phase genes. Therefore, in G_1, pRb appears to act as a cell cycle suppressor by binding members of the E2F transcription factor family. In retinoblastoma and several other tumours, pRb is absent or inactive, and cells passage through the G_1–S checkpoint unchecked (Ch. 43).

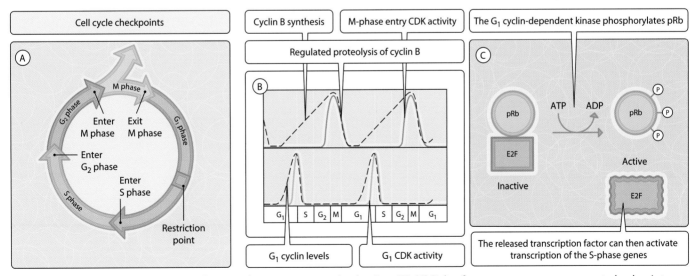

Fig. 3.41.2 Checkpoints in the cell cycle (A) and triggers to pass checkpoints (B). (C) Role of tumour suppressor genes at checkpoints.

42. DNA replication

Questions
- How is DNA synthesis achieved against the two DNA strands?
- How does a cell ensure rapid replication of its genome during cell division?
- How may nucleotide analogues interrupt the cell cycle?

Replication of strands

During S phase (6–8 h), each of the 46 chromosomes are replicated to form a sister chromatid joined to the original molecule through the centromere. DNA replication commences at specific origin-of-replication sites with ATP-dependent unwinding of the chromatin structure by DNA helicase to expose binding sites for a priming RNA polymerase. DNA topoisomerase also acts to break and rejoin the unwound strands to prevent tangling of the structure through super-coiling. Single-stranded-DNA-binding protein binds to the unwound strands to protect them from degradation before DNA duplication begins. One of the unwound strands will have 3′–5′ polarity (leading strand) and the other will have 5′–3′ polarity (lagging strand) Because DNA polymerase only catalyses synthesis in the 5′–3′ direction, a different process is required for the lagging strand.

Replication against the 3′–5′ leading strand
Initiation requires the 5′–3′ synthesis of a small RNA fragment (10–20 nucleotides) against the template strand (leading strand) reading in the 3′ to 5′ direction (Fig. 3.42.1, top). This is catalysed by specific RNA polymerases or primases that do not require priming oligonucleotides. Using the RNA fragment as primer, DNA polymerase III then catalyses the efficient incorporation of base-paired nucleotides against the leading strand and the elongation reaction that forms the sister chain in the 5′-3′ polarity. Thus, at each origin of replication site two DNA polymerase complexes can bind and two replication forks are generated, which move away from each other as synthesis proceeds.

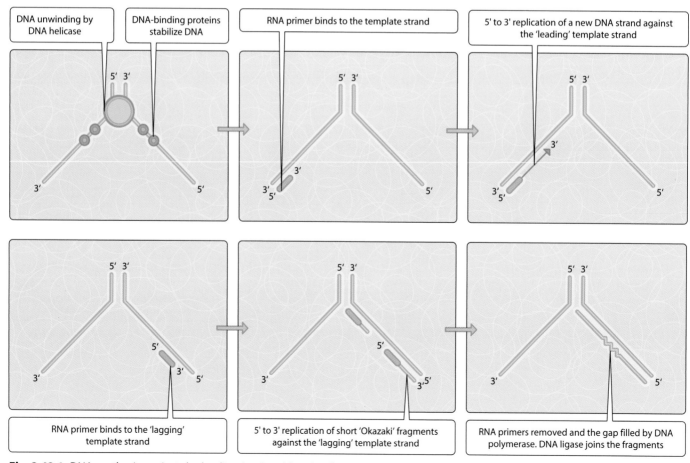

Fig. 3.42.1 DNA synthesis against the leading (top) and lagging (bottom) strands.

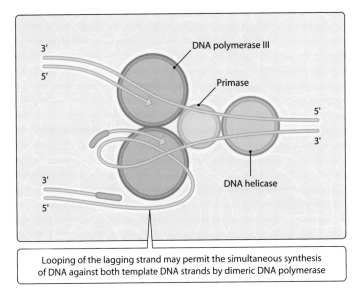

Looping of the lagging strand may permit the simultaneous synthesis of DNA against both template DNA strands by dimeric DNA polymerase

Fig. 3.42.2 Simultaneous synthesis of leading and lagging DNA strands.

Replication against the 5'–3' lagging strand

Synthesis against the other parental strand (5'–3' lagging strand) must occur in the opposite direction (Fig. 3.42.1, bottom). DNA duplication on the lagging strand is by a different discontinuous mechanism and produces short fragments ($\approx$ 1000 nucleotides) of new DNA, termed Okazaki fragments. As on the leading strand, duplication is initiated by synthesis of an RNA primer, which directs synthesis of DNA by DNA polymerase III. This occurs until the polymerase meets the initiating RNA primer of the preceding segment of DNA sequence, resulting in an Okazaki fragment. It has been proposed that dimeric DNA polymerase acts on a looped DNA structure at each replication fork so that DNA synthesis occurs on both strands essentially simultaneously (Fig. 3.42.2). To complete the new DNA strand

generated against the lagging strand, the short sections of priming RNA are removed by a 5'–3' RNAase H. DNA polymerase I completes the DNA strand in the gap and adjacent DNA fragments are then joined by a DNA ligase driven by hydrolysis of ATP or by NAD^+ (some prokaryotes).

Replicons

To ensure that the whole genome is replicated within the short time period of S phase, multiple replication forks are activated in clusters (up to 100) on each chromosome. These move in opposite directions from adjacent origin-of-replication sites meeting eventually over termination sites where adjacent segments of new DNA are ligated. The length of DNA produced between two origins is approximately the same as that required by one loop of the chromatin structure or a single gene and is termed a replicon (up to 300 000 base pairs) (Fig. 3.42.3).

DNA REPLICATION INHIBITORS IN CANCER THERAPY

Disruption of the supply of any of the four nucleotides for DNA synthesis leads to interruption of the cell cycle in S phase. This is the basis of anticancer therapies using drugs such as 5-fluorouracil and methotrexate, which block the synthesis of dTTP. Such treatments target any rapidly dividing cells, which include tumour cells. Other rapidly dividing tissues such as progenitor blood cells, gut epithelium, skin and hair follicles are also affected and lead to major unwanted effects: anaemia, sickness and hair loss. In particular, patients become immunosuppressed owing to drug-induced neutropenia and may become platelet depleted, leading to increased risk of bruising and haemorrhage.

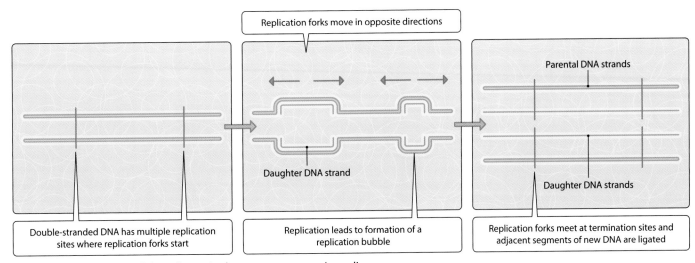

Replication forks move in opposite directions

Parental DNA strands

Daughter DNA strand

Daughter DNA strands

Double-stranded DNA has multiple replication sites where replication forks start

Replication leads to formation of a replication bubble

Replication forks meet at termination sites and adjacent segments of new DNA are ligated

Fig. 3.42.3 Replication of the eukaryotic chromosome occurs in replicons.

43. Cell cycle arrest

Questions
- Why is cell cycle arrest important?
- What are the main mechanisms of DNA repair?
- How may errors in cell cycle arrest lead to cancer?

The cell cycle may be arrested at two points (G_1–S and G_2–M) as a result of DNA damage (Figs 3.43.1 and 3.43.2). Mechanisms of cell cycle arrest involve inhibition of regulation of cyclin-dependent protein kinases (CDKs) by phosphorylation or CDK inhibitors. For example, the tumour suppressor gene product p53 is important in arresting the cell cycle at G_1, thereby preventing the replication of damaged DNA, and it may stimulate DNA repair indirectly. Expression of p53 is normally low but is increased dramatically when cell DNA is damaged, leading to the suggestion that it is a 'guardian of the genome'. p53 induces the expression of the CDK inhibitor p21, which inhibits G_1–S CDK.

DNA repair
Maintaining the integrity of the genetic information carried by the DNA of an organism is vital to survival. In addition to depurination (loss of a purine base) and deamination (loss of an amine group from a base), which occur spontaneously (5000–10 000 and 100 times per genome per day, respectively), the cell must resist the effects of environmental agents such as chemical mutagens and physical forces (e.g. ultraviolet radiation, X-rays, cosmic radiation). Some damage is self-inflicted, the result of errors in replication, and there are specific mismatch repair enzymes that scan newly synthesized DNA to replace wrongly incorporated bases. Unrepaired damage can lead to mutation, loss of information and may even block replication. As a consequence, cells express several enzymes that have the task of repairing damaged DNA before it is replicated. Simple lesions, such as those caused by alkylation of bases (covalent modification by alkyl groups), may be reversed, while other lesions are removed and replaced with new DNA.

Reversal of damage
Alkylating agents, such as nitrosoureas and nitrogen mustards, add alkyl groups to guanine residues (and other bases to a lesser degree). These alkyl groups may be removed directly by alkyl transferase enzymes, thus reversing the damage.

Replacement of damaged bases
Deaminated bases are cleaved from the sugar–phosphate backbone by specific DNA glycosylases (Fig. 3.43.3). The resulting apurinic or apyrimidinic sites (along with those produced by spontaneous depurination) are recognized by specific AP

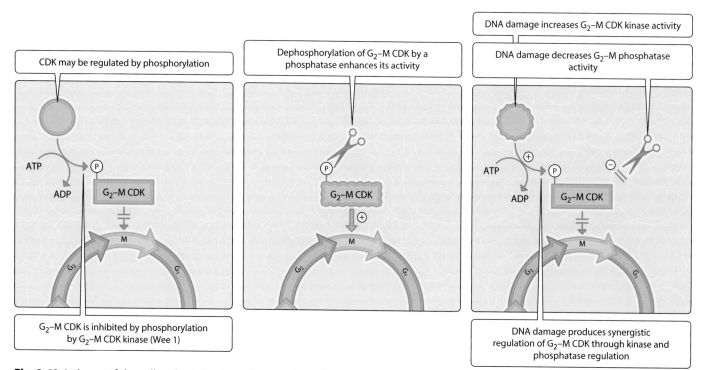

Fig. 3.43.1 Arrest of the cell cycle at G_2–M. CDK, cyclin-dependent protein kinase.

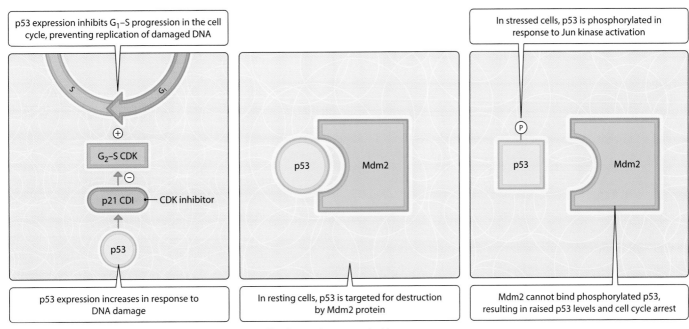

Fig. 3.43.2 Arrest of the cell cycle at G$_1$–S. CDK, cyclin-dependent protein kinase.

(apurinic or apyrimidinic) endonucleases, which nick the sugar–phosphate backbone next to the AP site. The damaged base can then be removed by an exonuclease and new DNA synthesized by DNA polymerase using the undamaged strand as template. The repair process is completed by DNA ligase, which seals the nick in the backbone. Larger lesions, such as the pyrimidine (cyclobutane) dimers produced by ultraviolet radiation, are corrected by excision repair, where a short stretch of the damaged strand is removed and replaced by new DNA.

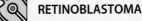 **RETINOBLASTOMA**

Mutation of the tumour suppressor gene *Rb* (the retinoblastoma susceptibility gene), which regulates passage through the G$_1$–S cell cycle checkpoint, results in retinal tumours in the young (Ch. 41). Both copies of *Rb* must be mutated for retinoblastoma to develop. In the more common inherited form, the patient inherits one defective and one wild-type *Rb* allele. Mutation in the wild-type allele, which has a high mutation rate, results in two defective alleles and usually the development of bilateral retinoblastoma at a young age.

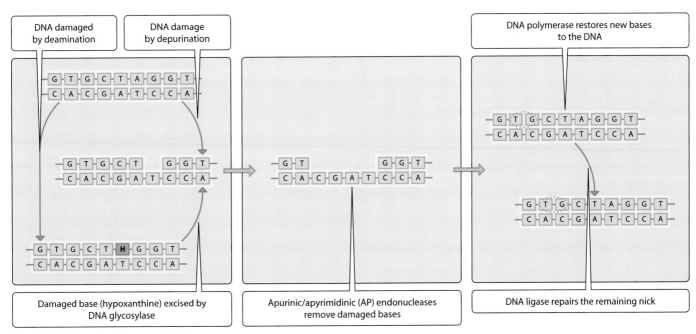

Fig. 3.43.3 Repair of damaged DNA.

44. Mitosis

Questions
- What is mitosis?
- What major anatomical changes are apparent in interphase, prophase, prometaphase, metaphase, anaphase, telophase and cytokinesis during the mitotic cycle?
- What is the genetic complement of daughter cells after mitosis?

Mitosis or M phase is a continuous dynamic process in vivo but can be subdivided into five mitotic stages (nuclear division) followed by a sixth stage of cytokinesis (cytoplasmic division) (Fig. 3.44.1). Mitosis is necessarily a highly accurate process to ensure the correct segregation of sister chromosomes. The result of mitotic cell division is the production of two daughter cells that contain a complete copy of the genome of the parent cell.

Prophase
As the cell moves from G_2 phase into prophase, the sister chromatids, duplicated during interphase, begin to condense into well-defined chromosomal structures and the nucleolus is disassembled. In the cytoplasm, the microtubular cytoskeletal network is also disassembled and reorganized on the surface of the nucleus to form the basis of the mitotic spindle. This structure is a bipolar arrangement of polar microtubules, which is capped at each end by a pair of centrioles, the mitotic centre (the centriole pair is duplicated during S phase), from which astral microtubules radiate. During prophase, the two centriole pairs, which begin lying side by side, are pushed away from each other by the growing bundles of polar microtubules forming the polar mitotic spindle.

Prometaphase
The disruption of the nuclear envelope into vesicular fragments signals the beginning of prometaphase. During this phase, microtubules associate with specialized points of attachment in the pericentriolar material on either side of the centromeres of condensed chromosomes called kinetochores. With the dissolution of the nuclear envelope, the kinetochore microtubules form initially random associations with the mitotic spindle and gradually orientate alongside the polar microtubular network. Then, by a series of jerky movements, the chromosomes are rearranged at right angles to the mitotic spindle (metaphase plate) so that the centromeres are aligned.

Metaphase
When the chromosomes are aligned at the centre of the mitotic spindle, the cell is said to be in metaphase. Each chromosome is held in position at the metaphase plate by the kinetochore microtubules attached to the paired kinetochores. This phase appears as a period of relative inactivity during nuclear division and can last a relatively long time.

Anaphase
In anaphase, the centromere splits in two, the paired kinetochores separate and the sister chromosomes migrate towards the opposite poles of the mitotic spindle. The kinetochore microtubules are seen to shorten as the chromosomes migrate towards the poles; at the same time, the polar microtubules elongate, increasing the separation between the poles of the spindle. Chromosomes are, therefore, pulled towards the mitotic poles, while the poles themselves are pushed apart. This phase often starts abruptly and lasts only a few minutes.

Telophase
Telophase marks the end of nuclear division. The kinetochore microtubules disassemble completely and the polar microtubules elongate still further before the mitotic spindle finally dissociates at the end of nuclear division. During this phase, the nuclear membrane reforms, the chromosomes begin to decondense into the dispersed chromatin structure and nucleoli begin to reform in the daughter nuclei.

Cytokinesis
The division of the cytoplasm is achieved by the formation of an actin microfilament ring under the plasma membrane at right angles to the mitotic spindle in the region of the cell corresponding to the position of the metaphase plate. Contraction of this structure commences usually in late anaphase to form a cleavage furrow. The cleavage furrow deepens progressively until the opposing edges meet and membrane fusion results in the completed division of the two daughter cells. Formation of the cleavage furrow may be arrested for a while if it meets residual mitotic spindle structures to form a midbody.

 INHIBITORS OF MITOSIS IN CANCER THERAPY

Treatment of mitotic cells with antimitotic, anticancer drugs such as colchicine, vinblastine and vincristine, which disrupt microtubule assembly, causes the disappearance of the mitotic spindle and blocks the cells in metaphase. By contrast, taxol causes mitotic arrest by stabilizing the mitotic spindle.

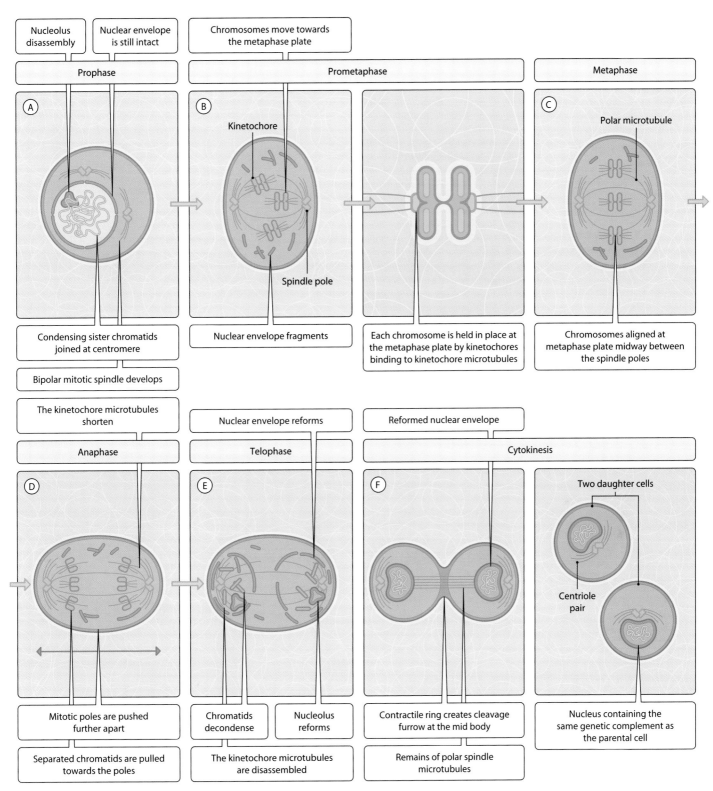

Fig. 3.44.1 Mitosis.

45. Meiosis

Questions
- What is meiosis?
- What are the differences between the first and second meiotic divisions
- What is the genetic complement of daughter cells after meiosis?

Meiosis is a specialized form of cell division that produces four genetically distinct haploid cells (containing only a single copy of each chromosome) from a diploid progenitor cell (containing two copies of each chromosome). This reductive form of cell division is found only in gamete production; in oogenesis and spermatogenesis. There are many similarities to mitotic cell division but also some important differences. Unlike mitosis, meiosis requires two rounds of cell division. The first round generates genetic variation (Fig. 3.45.1) and the second round produces haploid cells (Fig. 3.45.2). As in mitosis, meiosis can be divided into several stages.

First meiotic division
Interphase
Before the first meiotic cell division, the chromosomes of the diploid parental cell are replicated to form sister chromatids joined at the centromere.

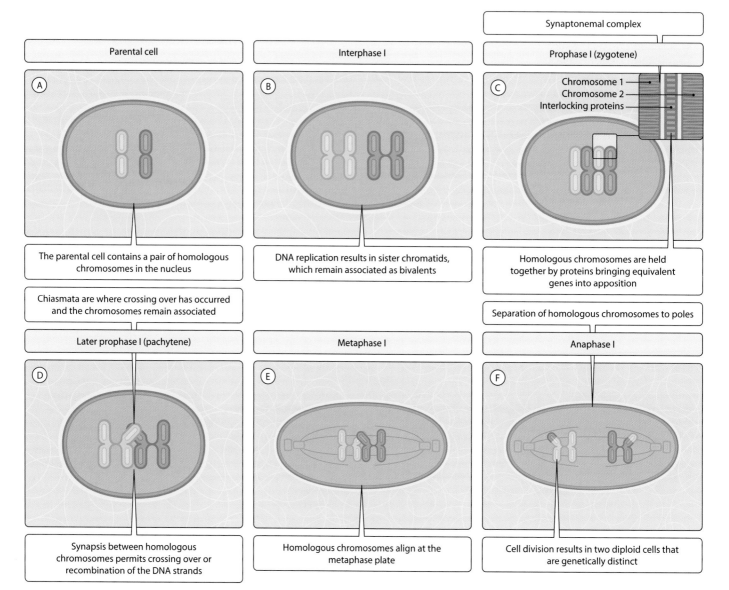

Fig. 3.45.1 Meiosis division 1.

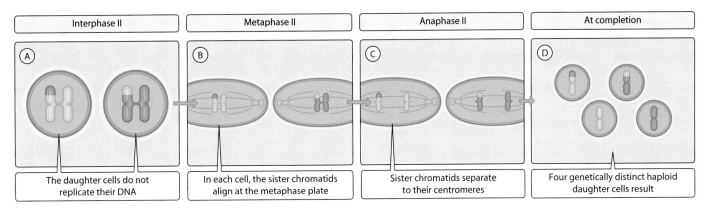

Interphase II	Metaphase II	Anaphase II	At completion
Ⓐ	Ⓑ	Ⓒ	Ⓓ
The daughter cells do not replicate their DNA	In each cell, the sister chromatids align at the metaphase plate	Sister chromatids separate to their centromeres	Four genetically distinct haploid daughter cells result

Fig. 3.45.2 Meiosis division 2.

Prophase I

On entering the first round of division, the sister chromatids, which remain associated (bivalents), condense into long thin strands stabilized by a central protein axis. As prophase continues, homologous chromosomes form closely associated pairs, synapses, along their entire length, bringing equivalent genes into apposition. The condensing structure forms a ladder-like proteinaceous axis from the two contributing chromosomes against which the chromatids are aligned, termed the synaptonemal complex. When the synapsis is complete, a period of recombination or crossing-over occurs (**pachytene**) where segments of paired maternal and paternal DNA can be exchanged between homologous chromosomes, resulting in increased genetic variation in the germ cell lines. On average, two to three cross-over events occur per pair of chromosomes. The two homologous chromosomes in a bivalent then decondense; however, as they move away from each other they remain associated at points at which cross-over events have taken place, **chiasmata**. RNA synthesis may occur against the unravelling chromatids. This is important for the production of storage material during the development of oocytes (eggs). In the late part of this phase (diakenesis), the chromosomes condense and each bivalent is observed to contain four chromatids, with sister chromatids joined at the centromere and non-sister chromatids joined at the chiasmata. The nuclear envelope breaks down, releasing the condensed chromosomes to interact with the completed spindle structure. Prophase I is the longest stage in meiotic cell division and completion of the first division and the whole of the second division may only take 10% of the time spent in prophase I.

Metaphase I

In metaphase I, the synaptic pairs of chromosomes move to the equator of the cell and orientate at right angles to the spindle.

Although non-identical, the X and Y sex chromosomes also pair owing to a region of similarity within their structure.

Anaphase I

Unlike the mitotic anaphase, the sister chromatids remain associated by the centromeres. Instead, the homologous synaptic pairs separate towards opposite poles of the spindle. The result of the first nuclear division is two diploid cells that are genetically distinct because of the independent assortment of parental chromosomes and recombination events.

The second meiotic division

The interphase between the first and second meiotic cell divisions does not involve DNA replication and differs, therefore, from the first meiotic division and mitosis. In other ways, the second meiotic cell division is analogous to mitosis. The sister chromatids separate at their centromeres during anaphase II and segregate to the opposite spindle pole. The result of meiotic cell division is the production of four cells that contain non-identical haploid copies of the genome.

 NUMERICAL CHROMOSOME ABNORMALITIES

Abnormalities in the chromosome complement in all cells of the body can occur through the failure of chromosomes to separate properly during meiotic cell division. This condition is lethal when a pair of chromosome homologues is missing (nullisomy) and when one chromosome is missing (monosomy). Usually the presence of one extra chromosome (trisomy) is also lethal but rare examples may survive to term. Patients with Down's syndrome (trisomy 21) may survive into adulthood.

46. Fertilization

Questions
- How do oocyte and sperm interact to begin the process of fertilization?
- What are the functions of Ca^{2+} in the fertilization process?
- When do maternal and paternal chromosomes first mix after fertilization?
- What methods are available to assist conception?

Gametes
In the male, the four haploid cells produced by meiosis go on to develop into spermatozoa (Fig. 3.46.1), with very little cytoplasm, a nucleus containing condensed chromatin and a motile flagellum. In females, meiosis is halted in prophase I to allow for yolk production (Fig. 3.46.2) in the primary oocyte. The secondary oocyte is arrested again at metaphase II and the second meiotic division is only completed if the egg is fertilized.

Fusion of egg and sperm
The fusion of egg and sperm at fertilization and the mixing of their haploid genomes restores the diploid genotype. As sperms swim through the female reproductive tract, they undergo an unknown process of capacitation, which permits them to fuse with an oocyte. Fusion begins via species-specific interactions with glycoproteins in the zona pellucida of the oocyte. A massive influx of Ca^{2+} is triggered in the **acrosome reaction** (Fig. 3.46.3), which induces the release of hydrolytic enzymes from the acrosome vesicle of the sperm to digest the zona pellucida and allow the sperm to penetrate to the plasma membrane of the oocyte. Polymerization of actin in the sperm head results in an extension of an acrosomal process and the sperm and oocyte plasma membranes fuse when they meet. Fusion stimulates the immediate release of cortical granules from the oocyte containing enzymes that modify the zona pellucida to prevent penetration of further sperm; the sperm nucleus enters the egg and there is a dramatic rise in $[Ca^{2+}]_i$ from the release of intracellular Ca^{2+} stores. This stimulates the progression of meiosis from metaphase II in the secondary oocyte while the male chromosomes remain isolated within a pronucleus. After meiosis is completed, mixing of the maternal and paternal chromosomes in the zygote first occurs during the metaphase of the first mitotic division.

Assisted conception
Several methods of assisted conception have been developed for the treatment of infertility. In gamete intrafallopian transfer (GIFT), ova are collected and delivered to the oviduct laparoscopically. Partner or donor sperm is delivered at the same time and fertilization takes place in the Fallopian tube. This procedure can be used where ovulation is impaired, for moderate sperm dysfunction or where there are problems with sperm transport in the female tract. Fertilization may also be achieved in vitro by mixing ova and sperm in a test tube. In this case, only fertilized ova are selected for replacement and ova containing three or more pronuclei are discarded as this indicates fusion

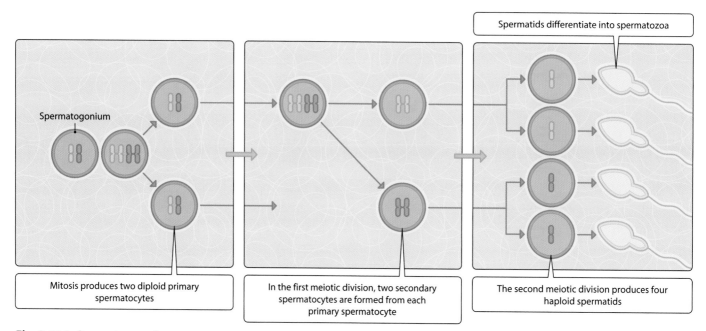

Spermatids differentiate into spermatozoa

Spermatogonium

Mitosis produces two diploid primary spermatocytes

In the first meiotic division, two secondary spermatocytes are formed from each primary spermatocyte

The second meiotic division produces four haploid spermatids

Fig. 3.46.1 Spermatogenesis.

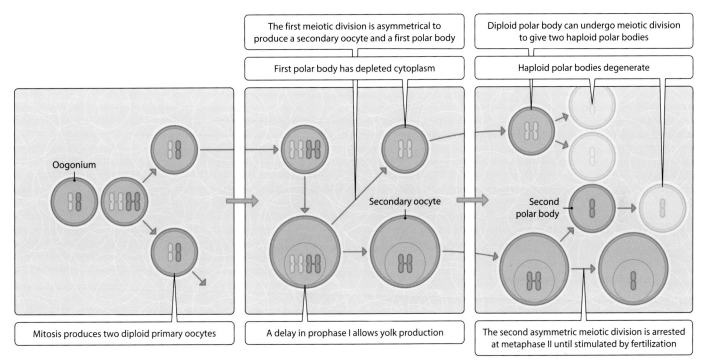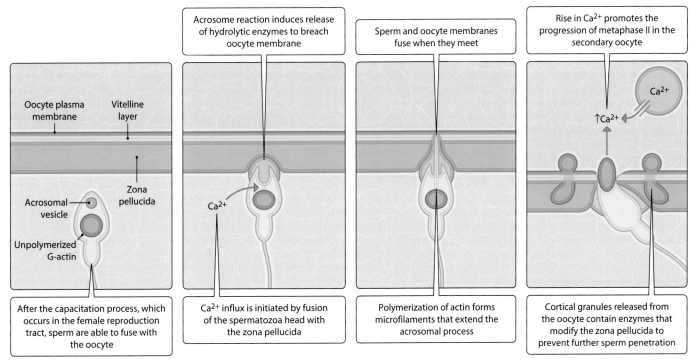

with two or more sperm. In vitro fertilization is indicated particularly when Fallopian tubes are blocked. If there is severe sperm dysfunction, fertilization may be achieved by intracytoplasmic sperm injection (ICSI). In this technique, a single sperm is injected directly into an ovum selected to be in metaphase II. Interestingly, the acrosome reaction is bypassed by this procedure but injected ova still develop into normal zygotes. In some cases of severe male infertility (e.g. round-headed sperm (globozospermia)), fertilization does not occur at high frequency even after ICSI, suggesting that additional factors are provided by the sperm to permit fertilization. It is also worth consideration that, although ICSI presents the only opportunity for conception to some infertile males, genetic defects in sperm production will be passed on to the next generation.

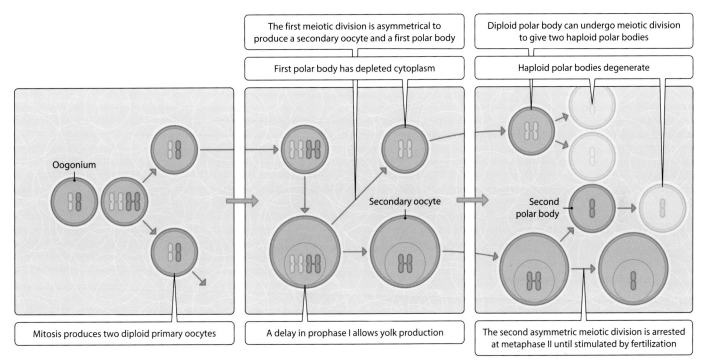

Fig. 3.46.2 Oogenesis.

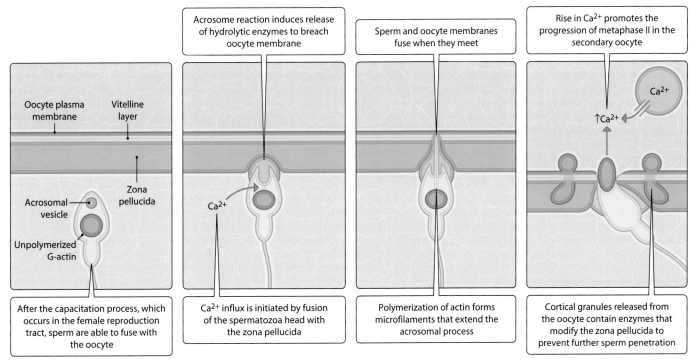

Fig. 3.46.3 Fusion of sperm and egg: the acrosome reaction.

47. Cancer

Questions
- What is the difference between an oncogene and a proto-oncogene?
- In what ways do oncogenes lead to tumourigenesis?
- Why do cells become cancerous?

A cancer is an uncontrolled growth and division of cells that have escaped the normal regulatory mechanisms of the cell cycle. Cancerous or tumour or neoplastic cells are said to be transformed. Transformed cells characteristically continue to divide under conditions in which normal cells would become quiescent (i.e. with contact inhibition or when nutrients or growth factors are depleted from the medium). A cancer is said to be benign when the growth is localized to the site of origin within a tissue, with no invasion, and malignant when the tumour cells can invade into the surrounding tissue and vasculature, spread to distant sites and grow there forming secondary tumours (**metastasis**).

Tumourigenesis: the somatic cell theory of cancer
Cancers arise because of mutations in the genome of somatic cells as a result of inaccuracies in gene replication or chromosomal rearrangement at mitosis (Fig. 3.47.1). If a result of the mutation is loss of control of cell growth and division, the mutant cell divides more rapidly than the surrounding tissue to form a clone of daughter tumour cells. Tumourigenesis is complex and requires more than one somatic mutation before full transformation of the cell occurs. Such a multistage process may occur over a period of years, with contributory mutations being accumulated over many generations of the cell (Fig. 3.47.2). Although the origin of cancer is genetic, it is not usually a hereditary disease. It is noteworthy that some rare familial predispositions to cancer are known. The somatic cell theory explains why cancers are not seen often in young people and why the incidence of cancer increases with age in the population.

Tumourigenic mutations most often arise because of inaccuracies in DNA replication, hereditary deficiencies in DNA repair and exposure to radiation or chemical carcinogens. Radiation (X-rays, γ-rays and ultraviolet light) may induce tumourigenic mutations by direct damage of the DNA or indirectly through errors arising during subsequent DNA repair by the cell. The mutagenic action of many carcinogens is not known but some act by intercalating in double-stranded DNA and disrupting normal structure, thereby affecting DNA replication. Carcinogens may themselves be mutagens or may be processed in the liver into an active mutagenic form.

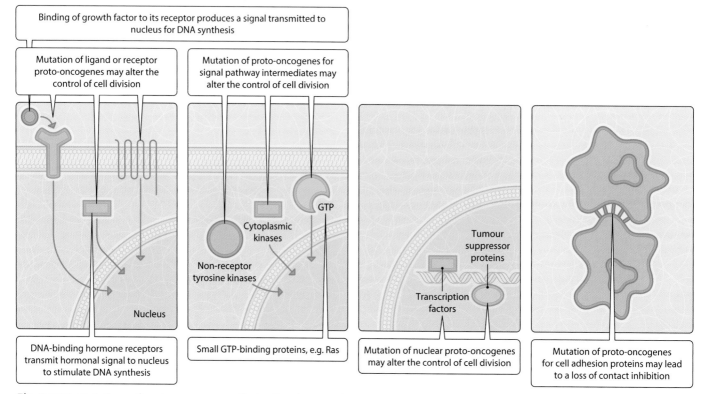

Fig. 3.47.1 Mutations of proto-oncogenes affect cell cycle control.

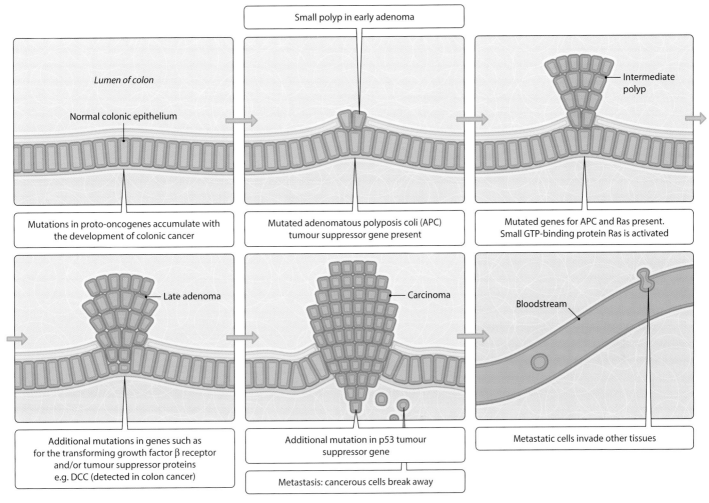

Fig. 3.47.2 Development of colonic cancer.

Viruses and tumourigenesis

Viral infection of cells is associated with several human cancers. All of the tumour viruses insert their genome into that of the host for replication and thereafter are reproduced in daughter cells. Tumourigenesis results either from the disruption of the structure and/or expression of a local host cell gene or **proto-oncogene**, a process known as insertional mutagenesis, or from the expression of virally encoded genes, **oncogenes**, which are responsible directly for the transformation of the cell.

Oncogenes and proto-oncogenes

Oncogenes were discovered as virally encoded genes that resulted in the loss of host cell growth control when expressed in virus-invaded cells. The proteins encoded by oncogenes are related to the products of non-oncogenic cellular genes, termed proto-oncogenes. These potentially oncogenic genes have important functions in normal cells, either in signalling and/or the regulation of cell differentiation. Their oncogenic potential arises from their ability to mimic signal pathway components or transcription factors, which ultimately lead to a modified control of key regulatory genes.

The presence of oncogenes in viral genomes probably occurred through recombination of an ancestral viral genome with proto-oncogenes in the host cell followed by subsequent mutation into an active oncogene. Expression of cellular oncogenes or the abnormal expression of proto-oncogenes is thought to override normal cell cycle control and lead to uncontrolled cell proliferation. This is clearly an advantage for the virus, which makes use of the host cell machinery for its replication.

Tumour suppressor genes

In normal cells, the activity of tumour suppressor genes is anti-oncogenic (Ch. 43). Loss of activity results in constitutive activation of cell growth.

48. Free radicals and oxidative damage

Questions
- What are free radicals and how are they produced?
- What protective mechanisms may be employed by cells to protect themselves from the damaging effects of free radicals?
- How may free radicals contribute to disease processes?

Free radicals in normal cell function

A free radical is any molecule that contains an atom with an unpaired electron. They are produced by oxidation/reduction reactions where there is transfer of single electrons only or when a covalent bond is broken leaving a single electron with each atom. Free radicals are highly reactive. The presence of the unpaired electron in the valence shell renders the atom highly unstable, such that either donation or receipt of an electron, as appropriate, is favoured to stabilize the shell.

Many free radicals are produced in cells during normal metabolism (Fig. 3.48.1). A particularly rich source is the electron transport system in mitochondria. Electrons that leak from the respiratory chain reduce molecular oxygen (O_2) directly to the superoxide anion ($O_2^{\bullet-}$). In addition, enzymes involved in other processes, such as detoxification (e.g. cytochrome P450), catecholamine neurotransmitter breakdown (e.g. monoamine oxidase) and cell signalling (e.g. nitric oxide synthase) also produce free radicals as part of their normal function. In some cases, free radicals are indispensable to normal cellular function: some enzymes catalyse the conversion of substrates into transient free radical species during their reaction mechanism (nitric oxide synthase). The hypochorite ion (OCl^-) is produced by myeloperoxidase in neutrophils to kill engulfed pathogens.

Because they are so reactive, free radicals react with all types of molecule including DNA, protein, lipid and carbohydrate, often producing damaging modifications. The products of reaction with free radicals are often free radicals themselves and, hence, damaging cascades of reactions can be set up. Normally, cells are protected from excessive free radical damage through the presence of dietary free radical scavengers or antioxidants (e.g. vitamins C and E). In addition, cells protect themselves against free radical damage by the expression of a variety of enzymes (e.g. catalase, superoxide dismutase) and the production of redox active chemicals (e.g. glutathione).

Problems arise for cells when levels of free radicals exceed protective mechanisms. Raised production can occur in response to exposure to ionizing radiation (e.g. sunlight, medical X-rays), chemicals (e.g. chlorine, ozone, nitrous oxide, cigarette smoke, alcohol, unsaturated fats and heavy metals) and even after strenuous physical activity and emotional stress.

Free radicals in disease

Radicals based on oxygen (e.g. superoxide anion, $O_2^{\bullet-}$, hydroxyl, $OH^\bullet$, hyperchlorite, OCl^-) and related highly oxidizing singlet oxygen (O^-) and hydrogen peroxide (H_2O_2) are known collectively as 'reactive oxygen species' (ROS) and are implicated in ageing and disease processes such as atherosclerosis, cancer, cataracts, diabetes mellitus, heart disease, ischaemia–reperfusion injury, neurodegeneration and rheumatoid arthritis.

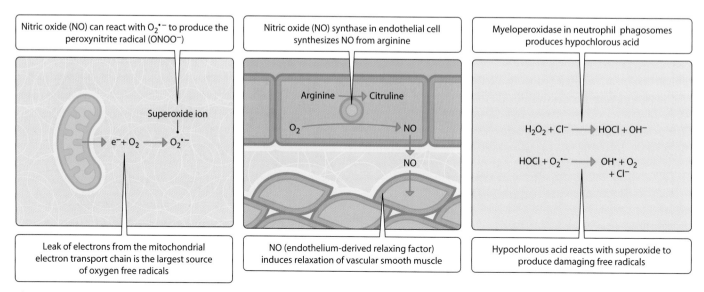

Fig. 3.48.1 Production of free radicals.

Thousands of oxidative reactions occur between ROS and DNA in each human cell every day. While the majority of these damaging events are repaired, accumulations of detrimental modifications that result in loss of function of the gene product over a lifetime contribute to the process of ageing. Similarly, ROS-mediated modification of proto-oncogenes may contribute to tumourigenesis (Ch. 47). ROS-mediated oxidation of membrane phospholipids disrupts membrane integrity.

ATHEROSCLEROSIS

In atherosclerosis, low density lipoproteins (LDL) accumulate within vessels with damaged endothelia, where blood flow is low (Fig. 3.48.2). Oxidative damage of LDL by ROS renders them unrecognizable by normal LDL receptors. Instead, they are recognized by scavenger receptors on macrophages, which accumulate large amounts to become foam cells and the beginnings of an atherosclerotic plaque.

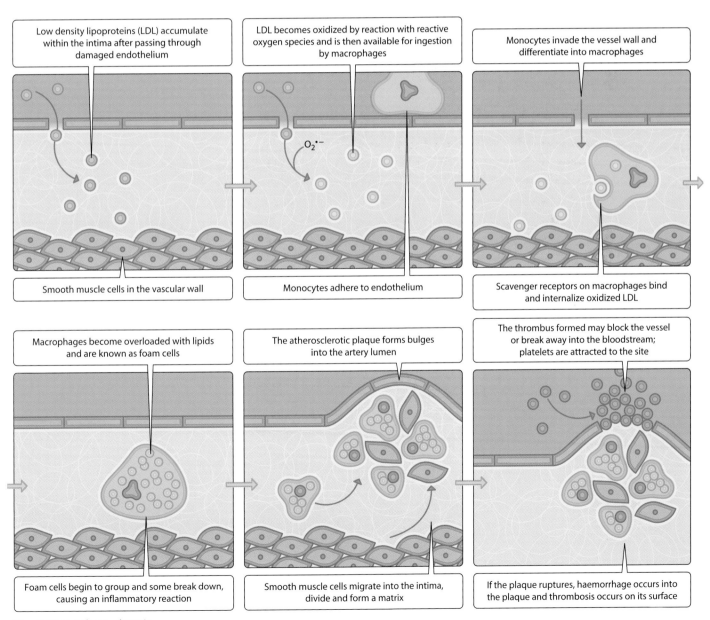

Fig. 3.48.2 Atherosclerosis.

49. Apoptosis

Questions
- What is necrosis?
- What is apoptosis?
- How does apoptosis contribute to tissue physiology?
- How can cells undergoing apoptosis be distinguished from necrotic cells?

Necrosis and apoptosis

Two types of cell death can be distinguished: necrosis and apoptosis (Fig. 3.49.1). 'Accidental' cell death or necrosis occurs after severe and sudden injury. It is characterized by the swelling of organelles and a breakdown of the integrity of the plasma membrane, which results in the leakage of cellular contents and an inflammatory response. Programmed cell death or apoptosis occurs in response to physiological triggers in development (tissue remodelling), defence, homeostasis and ageing. Apoptotic cells initially shrink; the cytoskeleton and nuclear envelope break down and the cells lose microvilli and cell junctions. Organelles maintain their structure but the plasma membrane becomes highly convoluted and the cell breaks down into small apoptotic bodies, which are quickly phagocytosed by macrophages. This occurs without leakage of cellular constituents and, hence, without an inflammatory response. Apoptosis is often accompanied by a characteristic condensation and fragmentation of chromatin by endogenous endonuclease activity between centrosomes.

Mechanisms of programmed cell death

The activation of proteolytic enzymes called **caspases** from inactive procaspases is central to the apoptotic process. Activation of the proteolytic caspase cascade occurs in response to extracellular or intracellular death signals, which result in the

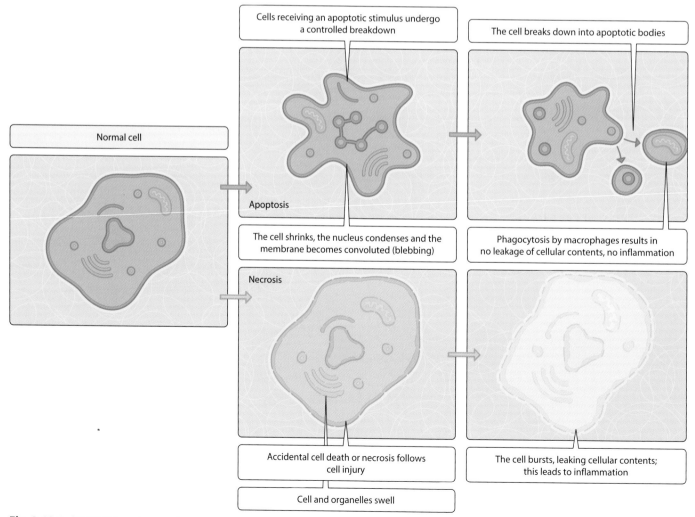

Fig. 3.49.1 Apoptosis and necrosis.

aggregation and activation of procaspase enzymes on intracellular adaptor proteins. Raised $[Ca^{2+}]_i$ and increased mRNA and protein synthesis, including that from cell cycle regulatory genes, proto-oncogenes (e.g. c-*myc*, c-*fos* and c-*jun*) and tumour suppressor genes (e.g. *p53*), are commonly, but not universally, implicated in apoptosis. Whether implicated gene products induce cell proliferation or apoptosis probably depends on their associations with other proteins and reflects the complexity and fine balance of the regulation of the cell cycle.

Several important molecular candidates are implicated in the apoptotic process.

- Fas ligand: released by stressed cells, on binding to the death factor receptor Fas, leads to recruitment of adaptor proteins and the aggregation and activation of caspase-8 (Fig. 3.49.2A).
- Cytochrome *c*: released from mitochondria in stressed cells and triggers activation of a caspase cascade via the adaptor protein (Apaf-1) (Fig. 3.49.2C).
- p53: DNA damage induces the production of p53, a transcription factor that results in the arrest of the cell cycle in G_1 to allow DNA repair; should repair fail, p53 may trigger cell removal by apoptosis.
- Bcl-2 family of proteins: some family members (Bcl-2, Bcl-X_L) suppress some apoptotic pathways (e.g. mitochondrial cytochrome *c* release) and a reduction in Bcl-2 levels has been associated with apoptosis. Rather than acting as death inhibitors, other family members act as caspase activators and so promote cell death. Bax and Bak act to stimulate the release of cytochrome *c* from mitochondria, while Bad binds and inhibits Bcl-2 directly.

Cell senescence

As cells age they become senescent, that is they lose the ability to divide. This limits the maximum possible number of cell divisions and probably protects the organism from the accumulation of damaging somatic mutations. On successive cell divisions, repetitive DNA sequences that are found at the ends of chromosomes, called **telomeres**, become progressively shortened; consequently, they can act as markers of cell ageing. In germ cells, telomerase maintains the telomere length such that the organism does not become reproductively compromised.

APOPTOSIS IN DISEASE PROCESSES

Apoptosis plays important roles in many disease processes. An apoptotic response to DNA damage may protect tissues from viral infection. Apoptosis may be important in eliminating cells containing damaged DNA that could contribute to the initial development of cancer and in suppressing the neoplastic signals in others. Failure of apoptosis in these situations could contribute to the initiation of the tumourigenic process and the appearance of tumour cells resistant to cytotoxic therapy. Inappropriate induction of apoptosis may contribute significantly to degenerative diseases, and failure to deplete self-reactive T cells by apoptosis may be important in the development of autoimmune disease.

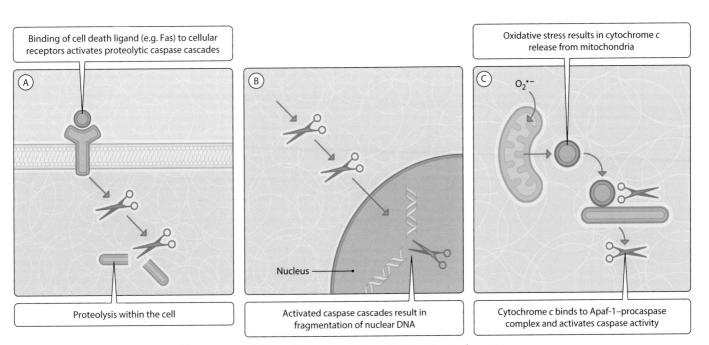

Fig. 3.49.2 Mechanisms involved in apoptosis: (A) Fas; (B) fragmentation of DNA; (C) cytochrome *c*.

50. Stem cells

Questions
- What are embryonic stem cells?
- Are adult cells terminally differentiated?
- How might the use of stem cells provide new therapies?

Differentiation

Although all new cells have the complete genome of the organism and, therefore, the genetic information necessary to differentiate to become any of the specialized cells of the body, most are already committed to a limited number of possible phenotypes. This has important implications for the processes of tissue renewal and repair. All humans develop from a single cell, the fertilized egg. Early embryos, called blastocysts, have an outer layer of protective support cells that encases a group of cells called totipotent embryonic stem cells (ESCs; Fig. 3.50.1). These cells, which are undifferentiated, have the potential to develop into any cell of the body. As the embryo develops further, these cells appear to become committed to one of three paths: **ectoderm** (giving rise to skin and neural tissue), **mesoderm** (blood, muscle and connective tissue) and **endoderm** (respiratory and digestive tissue). Differentiation into specialized, adult-type cells requires selective gene expression and exposure to specific hormonal and environmental cues.

Not all cells in an adult are fully committed to a particular fate. For example, blood cells (leukocytes and erythrocytes) are relatively short lived, being replenished by differentiation of progenitor cells produced from a common haemopoietic stem cell found in bone marrow. Stem cells are also found in other tissues; for example the epidermal layer of the skin is constantly being renewed as keratinocytes die and are lost from the surface.

Therapeutic approaches

Recently, the possibility of using ESCs to repair and regenerate damaged or diseased adult tissues has generated considerable excitement (Fig. 3.50.2). Could ESCs be used to repair damaged cardiac muscle after a heart attack or replace neural tissue lost by sufferers from, say, Parkinson's disease? Despite the potential offered by the plasticity of ESCs, there are significant challenges associated with such an approach. The use of embryonic tissue raises serious ethical issues and there is also the problem of overcoming rejection of the introduced cells. One possible solution to the problem of rejection, which has been approved in a small number of cases, is the creation of so-called 'designer siblings' to act as stem cell donors. These are children born from embryos that were chosen, by preimplantation genetic selection, for their compatibility with the intended recipient. A further, more radical, step would be the creation of embryos to provide compatible tissue grafts by reproductive cloning. While growth of a clone to produce fully developed organs would be ethically unacceptable, creation of an embryo to produce stem cells with self-antigens that could be seeded back into damaged tissue

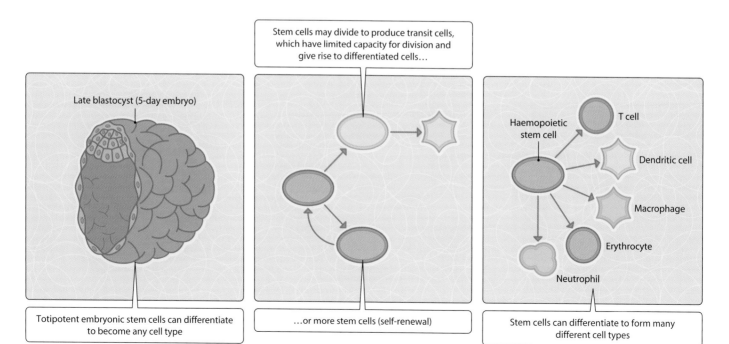

Late blastocyst (5-day embryo)

Stem cells may divide to produce transit cells, which have limited capacity for division and give rise to differentiated cells…

Haemopoietic stem cell

T cell

Dendritic cell

Macrophage

Erythrocyte

Neutrophil

Totipotent embryonic stem cells can differentiate to become any cell type

…or more stem cells (self-renewal)

Stem cells can differentiate to form many different cell types

Fig. 3.50.1 Stem cells.

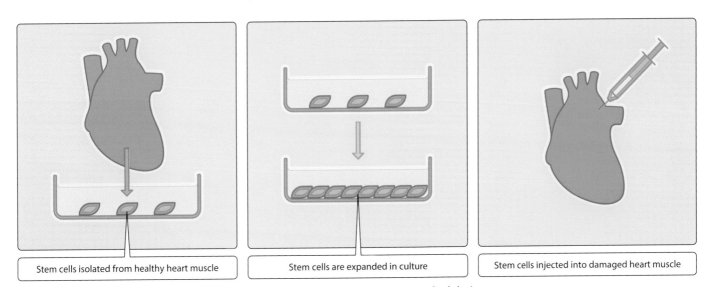

| Stem cells isolated from healthy heart muscle | Stem cells are expanded in culture | Stem cells injected into damaged heart muscle |

Fig. 3.50.2 Possible use of embryonic stem cells to repair and regenerate damaged adult tissues.

might be more likely to gain acceptance. In principle, haploid genetic material of a donated isolated oocyte is removed by aspiration and the diploid genetic material from a cell from the patient injected in its place. The conditions in the cytoplasm of the oocyte favour expression of the developmental genes of the diploid genome and cell division begins as if from a newly fertilized zygote. The resulting cells have the same surface antigens as the patient and so transplanted cells from the embryo should be recognized by the patient's immune system as self and not be rejected. The principle of reproductive cloning was proven with Dolly the sheep and similar developments in humans are likely to follow soon.

A more ethically acceptable alternative rests on the belief of some researchers that haemopoietic stem cells are capable of trans-differentiation, that is that they can become differentiated cells from different lineages, making them the perfect candidates for stem cell therapies, but this potential has yet to be demonstrated unequivocally.

It is accepted that stem cells exist in adult tissues with at least the potential to differentiate into one of a limited range of cell types (multipotent). Under normal circumstances, the replication of these cells must be tightly controlled otherwise tissue disruption will occur. The scientific challenge will include the identification and isolation of these cells and the development of an understanding of how they are regulated.

Stem cells and cancer

The apparently unlimited capacity of stem cells to renew themselves has parallels with the behaviour of cancer cells. This has led to speculation that at least some cancers could arise from mutation of adult stem cells. It has been suggested that it might require fewer mutations to cause a cell that already has replicative potential to escape from normal controls than would be required in the case of a terminally differentiated cell. The presence of small numbers of chemotherapy-resistant cancer stem cells in a mass of more differentiated cancer cells might explain why many drugs are capable of shrinking solid tumours but ultimately have little impact on prognosis as the tumour simply re-grows.

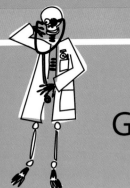

Glossary

Action potential
A brief, all-or-nothing change in potential across a cell membrane that propagates along the axon as a nerve impulse

Agonist
A substance that binds to a receptor and activates it

Antagonist
A substance that binds to a receptor and blocks its activity by preventing agonist binding

Apoptosis
Programmed cell death or cell suicide

Cell cycle
The time from one cell division to the next

Chromatin
A condensed form of a chromosome consisting of DNA and histone proteins

Codon
A sequence of three nucleotides (triplet) in messenger RNA that encodes an amino acid

Cytoskeleton
A complex framework of structural protein filaments forming a molecular scaffold that contributes to the shape and movement of a cell

Depolarization
A change in the potential across a cell membrane in an excitable cell whereby the inside of the cell becomes less negative relative to the outside than at the resting membrane potential

Desensitization (tachyphylaxis)
The process of reducing sensitivity of a cell to a continuing stimulus

Endocytosis
The uptake of extracellular solutes or particles by the formation of membrane vesicles by the inward folding (invagination) of the cell membrane

Endoplasmic (sarcoplasmic) reticulum
A network of membranous flattened sacs and tubules in the cytoplasm of a cell, involved in phospholipid and protein synthesis, Ca^{2+} storage and other functions

Eukaryote
An organism in which the cells contain a nucleus and other membrane-bound organelles

Exon
A segment within a gene encoding part of or a whole protein

Extracellular matrix
A mass of specialized proteins and polysaccharides found between cells

G-protein
A GTP-binding membrane-bound protein that acts as a molecular switch to transduce the information from a stimulated receptor to activate or inhibit an effector enzyme or ion channel

Golgi apparatus
A stack of flattened membranous sacs in which post-translational modification of newly synthesized proteins occurs

Homeostasis
The maintenance of a relatively constant internal environment

Hyperpolarization
A change in the potential across a cell membrane in an excitable cell whereby the inside of the cell becomes more negative relative to the outside than at the resting membrane potential

Intron
A non-coding segment within a gene

Ion channel
A membrane protein that permits ions to enter or leave a cell

Lysosome
A membrane-bound organelle that contains hydrolytic enzymes to break down cellular components

Meiosis
Reproductive cell division that produces four genetically distinct haploid cells (containing only a single copy of each chromosome) from a diploid progenitor cell (containing two copies of each chromosome)

Membrane
A phospholipid bilayer containing proteins that forms a semipermeable barrier around cells and organelles

Membrane potential
The electric potential that exists across a cell membrane; in a resting cell, it is negative inside relative to outside

Microtubules
Cytoskeletal protein filaments made up of linear polymers of tubulin

Mitochondrion
A double membrane-bound organelle that contains the enzymes of the Krebs cycle and fatty acid oxidation and carries out oxidative phosphorylation to produce most of the ATP in the cell

Mitosis
Somatic cell division that produces two diploid cells (containing two copies of each chromosome) from a diploid progenitor cell

Necrosis
Accidental cell death following cell injury

Nucleus
An organelle bound by a double membrane and containing the genetic material

Neurotransmitter
A chemical that relays electrical signals between a neuron and another cell

Oncogene
A gene that results in uncontrolled proliferation of a cell

Organelle
A membrane-bound structure within a cell that compartmentalizes cellular functions

Peroxisome
A membrane-bound organelle that segregates oxidative reactions involving molecular oxygen from other areas of the cell that they could damage

Phagocytosis
The internalization of receptor-bound virus, microorganism or particulate matter by phagocytic macrophages

Pinocytosis
The internalization of soluble substances by the formation of enclosed vesicles at the cell surface by endocytosis

Prokaryote
A cell or organism that lacks a membrane-bound nucleus

Proteasome
A multiprotein complex of protease enzymes that degrades unfolded and damaged proteins

Proto-oncogene
A normal gene that can mutate to a form which results in uncontrolled cell division and cancer

Receptor
A molecule on the surface or the inside of a cell that binds specifically to a messenger molecule to cause regulation of a cellular process

Ribosome
A complex macromolecular structure of ribosomal RNA and protein that directs protein synthesis from messenger RNA

Sarcomere
The smallest contractile unit of actin and myosin cytoskeletal proteins in striated muscle cells

Second messenger
A short-lived chemical signal generated in the cytosol in response to cell surface receptor activation that triggers a biochemical response; the second messenger can initiate an amplification cascade

Stem cell
An undifferentiated cell that can reproduce indefinitely and retains the potential to differentiate into many different mature cell types

Synapse
A specialized junction between excitable cells where nerve impulses are passed; usually mediated by a chemical messenger (neurotransmitter)

Transcription
The synthesis of a messenger RNA copy of a DNA (gene) template

Translation
The synthesis of a polypeptide chain against a messenger RNA template

Transporter
A membrane protein involved in the transmembrane movement of a solute

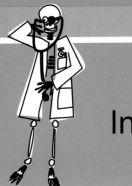

Index